HOLISTIC FAMILY HOME APOTHECARY

2500+ Ancient Natural Remedies and Step-by-Step Guides to Restore Health, Protect Your Family, and Achieve Lasting Family Wellness

Celia Mills

Table of Contents

Chapter 1: Foundations of Home Apothecary

Embarking on the journey to establish a holistic family home apothecary begins with understanding the core principles that have guided herbalists for centuries. At the heart of these principles lies the belief in the healing power of nature and the importance of living in harmony with the natural world. This foundational knowledge not only empowers individuals to care for their family's health naturally but also fosters a deep respect for the plants that support this wellness.

Selecting Quality Herbs and Ingredients

The efficacy of your home apothecary hinges on the quality of herbs and ingredients you choose. Opt for organically grown herbs to ensure they are free from pesticides and chemicals that can undermine their medicinal properties. When sourcing herbs, consider their origin, how they were grown, and the methods used for harvesting and drying. Freshness is also crucial; herbs should be vibrant in color and aroma, indicating their potency. For those unable to grow their own herbs, sourcing from reputable suppliers who provide detailed information about their products is essential.

Essential Tools for Your Home Apothecary

Equipping your home apothecary requires a selection of tools designed to aid in the preparation and storage of herbal remedies. Glass jars with tight-fitting lids are indispensable for storing dried herbs, tinctures, and salves, protecting them from light and air which can degrade their quality. A mortar and pestle, used for grinding herbs, allows for the release of their full medicinal properties. Additionally, a digital scale ensures precise measurements for recipes, crucial for maintaining consistency and effectiveness in your remedies.

Creating a Dedicated Space

Designating a specific area in your home for your apothecary promotes organization and efficiency. This space should be cool, dark, and dry to best preserve your herbs and preparations. Shelving that allows for easy categorization and access to your herbs, tools, and reference materials can streamline the preparation process. This dedicated space not only serves a practical function but also becomes a sanctuary for healing and learning.

By adhering to these foundational steps, you lay the groundwork for a home apothecary that is both functional and holistic. This approach not only ensures the preparation of effective natural remedies but also cultivates a lifestyle that values and incorporates the wisdom of herbal medicine into daily family life.

Understanding and Utilizing Herbal Properties

A crucial aspect of creating effective remedies in your home apothecary is a deep understanding of the properties and benefits of various herbs. Each herb possesses unique qualities that can address specific health concerns. For example, chamomile is renowned for its calming and anti-inflammatory effects, making it ideal for stress relief and digestive issues. Learning about these properties allows for the customization of remedies tailored to the specific needs of your family members.

Harvesting and Preparing Your Herbs

For those who choose to grow their own herbs, knowing when and how to harvest them is key to maximizing their medicinal value. Herbs should be harvested at the right time of day, typically in the morning after the dew has evaporated but before the sun is too intense, to ensure they retain their essential oils. The method of preparation also plays a significant role in the potency of the remedy. For instance, delicate herbs may require gentle drying or infusion to preserve their therapeutic properties, while tougher roots may need decoction, a process of boiling to extract their active compounds.

Storing Your Preparations

Proper storage of herbs and herbal preparations extends their shelf life and maintains their effectiveness. Dried herbs should be stored in airtight containers away from direct sunlight and moisture. Tinctures, which are alcohol or vinegar extractions of herbs, benefit from dark glass bottles to prevent light degradation. Labeling each container with the herb name, date of preparation, and expected shelf life helps in organizing your apothecary and ensures that you use the remedies within their optimal potency period.

Safety and Dosage Considerations

While natural remedies can offer significant health benefits, it is important to approach herbal medicine with an understanding of safety and appropriate dosages. Factors such as age, health condition, and possible interactions with other medications must be considered. Consulting with a healthcare professional knowledgeable in herbal medicine is advisable when starting out, especially when remedies are intended for children, pregnant women, or individuals with chronic health conditions.

Continued Learning and Experimentation

Building a holistic family home apothecary is an ongoing journey of learning and experimentation. Engaging with a community of herbalists, attending workshops, and reading extensively can enhance your knowledge and skills. Experimentation with creating your own remedies, such as soothing balms for skin irritations or herbal teas for relaxation, allows for personalization and a deeper connection with the healing power of herbs.

By integrating these practices into your home apothecary, you embrace a tradition of natural wellness that nurtures the health and well-being of your family. This hands-on approach to healthcare empowers you to take an active role in the healing process, grounded in the wisdom of herbal medicine and the bounty of nature.

Understanding Herbal Medicine

Herbal medicine, also known as phytotherapy, involves using plant-based materials for medicinal purposes. It is a practice rooted in every culture of the world and has a rich history that spans thousands of years. The basic premise of herbal medicine is that plants contain compounds that can affect the body's physiology in beneficial ways. To harness these effects, it is crucial to understand the active constituents of herbs, how they interact with the body, and how they can be safely and effectively used to address various health concerns.

Active Constituents of Herbs

Plants produce a wide range of chemical compounds, many of which have therapeutic effects. These include alkaloids, glycosides, flavonoids, and essential oils, among others. Each group of compounds has distinct properties and health benefits. For instance, alkaloids, found in herbs like echinacea and goldenseal, have immune-stimulating and antimicrobial effects. Flavonoids, present in chamomile and green tea, are known for their antioxidant and anti-inflammatory properties. Understanding these constituents is key to selecting the right herbs for specific health issues.

Herb-Body Interactions

The interaction between herbal compounds and the human body is complex. Herbs can act on the body in various ways, such as modulating the immune system, influencing hormone levels, or providing antimicrobial activity. The effect of an herb depends not only on its active constituents but also on the dosage, the method of preparation, and the individual's specific health conditions and constitution. For example, valerian root may act as a sedative and improve sleep quality in one individual, while it might have minimal effects on another, highlighting the importance of personalization in herbal therapy.

Methods of Preparation

The method of preparing an herb can significantly affect its therapeutic properties. Common preparations include teas, tinctures, capsules, and topical salves. Each method has its advantages and is chosen based on the desired outcome and the specific properties of the herb. Teas and decoctions are suitable for water-soluble compounds, whereas tinctures, which involve macerating herbs in alcohol or vinegar, are effective for extracting a wider range of constituents. Capsules offer convenience and precise dosing, while salves and balms are ideal for local application on the skin.

Safety Considerations

While herbal medicines are natural, they are not without risks. It is essential to consider safety aspects such as potential side effects, interactions with pharmaceutical medications, and contraindications. Certain herbs can interact with prescription drugs, either enhancing or inhibiting their effects, which can lead to adverse outcomes. Additionally, some herbs are contraindicated in specific conditions, such as pregnancy or in individuals with certain medical conditions. Therefore, a thorough understanding of an herb's safety profile is crucial before incorporating it into a treatment plan.

Quality and Sourcing of Herbs

The quality of herbal materials plays a critical role in their efficacy. Factors such as the plant's growing conditions, the timing of harvest, and the method of processing can all influence the potency of the final product. Sourcing herbs from reputable suppliers who provide detailed information about their products, including their origin and how they were grown and processed, ensures that you are using high-quality materials in your home apothecary.

By integrating a deep understanding of the principles of herbal medicine, including the active constituents of herbs, their interactions with the body, methods of preparation, safety considerations, and the importance of quality and sourcing, individuals can more effectively and safely use these natural remedies to support their health and well-being.

Dosage and Administration

Determining the correct dosage is paramount in herbal medicine to ensure safety and effectiveness. Unlike pharmaceuticals, herbal remedies can vary significantly in strength based on their source, preparation, and storage. Start with lower doses and adjust based on the individual's response, considering factors such as age, weight, and health status. For instance, tinctures might be administered in drops or milliliters, with specific guidelines provided for different age groups. Teas might be consumed in cups, with recommendations often suggesting one to three cups daily for adults. Always adhere to recommended dosages on commercial preparations or consult a professional when in doubt.

Personalization of Herbal Treatments

Herbal medicine shines in its capacity for personalization. Recognizing that each individual's body, health condition, and response to herbs can differ allows for tailored treatments. This personal approach starts with a thorough assessment of the person's health history, current medications, and specific health goals. For example, a calming herbal blend might be customized with additional herbs to support digestion if stress is contributing to gastrointestinal symptoms. This level of customization enhances the efficacy of herbal remedies and is a cornerstone of a holistic approach to health.

Integrating Herbs into Daily Life

Incorporating herbal remedies into daily routines can optimize health and prevent illness. This can range from adding immune-supporting herbs to your diet during cold and flu season to using adaptogenic herbs to manage stress. Simple practices, such as starting the day with a cup of herbal tea or using herbal-infused oils in cooking, can make herbal medicine a seamless part of everyday life. Additionally, creating rituals around the use of herbs, such as evening baths with relaxing herbal blends, can enhance their therapeutic benefits through the power of routine and intention.

Monitoring and Adjusting Treatments

Ongoing monitoring of the effects of herbal remedies is essential. Keep a journal to note any changes in symptoms or overall well-being. This record can be invaluable for adjusting treatments as needed, whether to increase the dose, try a different herb, or discontinue use. Listening to the body and being willing to modify the approach ensures that herbal treatments remain aligned with the individual's evolving health needs.

Engagement with Professional Guidance

While the home apothecary is a powerful tool for wellness, collaboration with healthcare professionals knowledgeable in both conventional and herbal medicine can enhance care. This partnership is particularly important for managing chronic conditions, navigating potential herb-drug interactions, and addressing complex health issues. Professionals can provide insights into the latest research, suggest specific herbal compounds, and offer guidance on safety and efficacy.

Building a Community of Herbal Enthusiasts

Joining or forming a community with others interested in herbal medicine can provide support, inspiration, and shared knowledge. Whether through local workshops, online forums, or study groups, connecting with fellow herbal enthusiasts encourages continuous learning and exchange of experiences. This community can be a valuable resource for discovering new herbs, preparation methods, and applications, further enriching the home apothecary experience.

By embracing these practices, individuals can deepen their understanding and application of herbal medicine, enhancing their health and well-being through the power of plants. The journey into herbal medicine is one of discovery, connection, and personal growth, offering a path to holistic health that is both empowering and rooted in ancient wisdom.

History and Philosophy of Natural Remedies

The roots of herbal medicine stretch deep into the fabric of human history, predating the written word and interwoven with the development of cultures across the globe. This ancient practice emerges from a universal human experience—the observation of nature and the recognition of its potent healing capabilities. The philosophy underpinning herbal medicine is grounded in the belief that the Earth provides all the necessary tools for healing. It's a philosophy that respects the intricate relationships between the human body, plant life, and the environment.

Cultural Traditions and Historical Use

Every civilization has its own tradition of using plants for medicinal purposes. From the **Ayurvedic** remedies of India, which utilize a comprehensive approach to health and wellness, focusing on balancing the body, mind, and spirit, to the **Traditional Chinese Medicine (TCM)** that employs an extensive pharmacopeia of herbs to restore balance and energy (Qi) within the body. In the Americas, indigenous tribes have relied on the vast biodiversity of their lands to treat ailments using herbal remedies passed down through generations. These traditions emphasize a holistic approach, viewing the individual as part of a larger whole—a concept that is central to herbal medicine.

Active Constituents and Synergy

Understanding the **active constituents** of herbs is crucial in herbal medicine. These are the chemical compounds within plants that have therapeutic effects on the human body. However, the philosophy of herbal medicine goes beyond the action of single constituents, embracing the idea of **synergy**—the concept that the therapeutic effect of the whole herb is greater than the sum of its parts. This holistic approach contrasts with the modern pharmaceutical model, which often isolates individual compounds. Herbalists argue that whole herbs bring a balance and a complexity that cannot be replicated in isolated chemicals.

The Doctrine of Signatures

An intriguing aspect of herbal philosophy is the **Doctrine of Signatures**, an ancient belief that plants resemble the parts of the body they are intended to treat. For example, the liverwort plant, with its liver-shaped leaves, was traditionally used to treat liver problems. While modern science doesn't support this theory as a basis for herbal efficacy, it highlights the historical effort to connect human health with the natural world, encouraging a deeper observation and respect for plant life.

Sustainability and Ethical Harvesting

The philosophy of herbal medicine also encompasses the principles of sustainability and ethical harvesting. With the growing interest in natural remedies, the importance of harvesting practices that ensure the longevity of plant species cannot be overstressed. Ethical wildcrafting—harvesting wild plants responsibly—protects biodiversity and respects the ecosystems from which these medicinal plants are drawn. This principle aligns with the broader philosophy of living in harmony with nature, recognizing that human health is deeply connected to the health of the planet.

Adaptation and Modern Integration

As herbal medicine transitions into the modern era, it faces the challenge of integrating ancient wisdom with contemporary scientific understanding. This integration involves rigorous scientific research to validate traditional uses of herbs, ensuring safety and efficacy for a wider acceptance in today's healthcare landscape. The growing body of research supports many traditional uses of herbs, offering a promising bridge between ancient practices and modern health needs.

Educational Empowerment

Central to the philosophy of herbal medicine is the empowerment of individuals to take charge of their own health. Through education and shared knowledge, herbal medicine demystifies healthcare, making it accessible and understandable. This empowerment fosters a proactive approach to health, encouraging individuals to maintain wellness through natural means and to understand their bodies on a deeper level.

Herbal medicine's rich tapestry of history and philosophy offers a profound perspective on health and healing. It invites us to reconsider our relationship with nature, urging a return to a more holistic, sustainable, and balanced approach to wellness. As we move forward, the integration of this ancient wisdom with modern science holds the potential to enrich our lives, offering pathways to health that are as nurturing to the planet as they are to our bodies.

Safety and Efficacy

Ensuring the safety and efficacy of herbal remedies is paramount in the holistic family home apothecary. This involves a meticulous approach to selecting, preparing, and administering herbs, grounded in an understanding of herbal properties and potential interactions. It's essential to recognize that while natural, herbs can have powerful effects on the body, necessitating a careful and informed approach to their use.

Identifying and Mitigating Potential Herb-Drug Interactions

One of the first steps in ensuring safety is to identify any potential interactions between herbal remedies and pharmaceutical medications. Certain herbs can either potentiate or inhibit the effects of drugs, leading to undesired outcomes. For instance, St. John's Wort, known for its antidepressant properties, can interact with a wide range of medications, including birth control pills, leading to decreased efficacy of these drugs. To mitigate such risks, thoroughly research each herb's interaction profile and consult with a healthcare professional before combining herbal remedies with pharmaceuticals.

Understanding Contraindications

Contraindications refer to conditions or scenarios where a particular herb should not be used. Many herbs are contraindicated during pregnancy and breastfeeding or in individuals with specific health conditions. For example, while echinacea is popular for immune support, it is generally recommended to avoid its use in progressive systemic and autoimmune disorders. Detailed knowledge of an herb's contraindications ensures that remedies are used safely, without inadvertently causing harm.

Administering Correct Dosages

Determining the correct dosage is critical for both safety and efficacy. Dosages can vary widely based on the herb, the form in which it's being used (tincture, tea, capsule, etc.), and the individual taking it. Factors such as age, body weight, and health status play a significant role in how an herb should be dosed. For example, the dosage of a valerian root tincture for promoting sleep in an adult will differ significantly from the dosage appropriate for a child. Utilize reputable sources and professional guidance to establish starting dosages and adjust as necessary based on response.

Quality Control and Herb Sourcing

The quality of herbs used in remedies significantly impacts their safety and efficacy. Herbs contaminated with pesticides, heavy metals, or adulterated with other, potentially harmful, plants can pose serious health risks. Prioritize sourcing herbs from reputable suppliers who test their products for purity and contaminants. Organic certification can be a reliable indicator of quality, though it's also valuable to know the supplier's practices regarding sustainable harvesting and fair trade.

Preparation and Storage Techniques

Proper preparation and storage of herbal remedies are vital to preserving their medicinal properties and preventing spoilage or contamination. Use non-reactive utensils and containers, such as glass or stainless steel, to avoid chemical reactions that could alter the remedy's effectiveness. Store dried herbs in airtight containers away from light and heat to maintain their potency. Tinctures and extracts should be kept in amber or dark glass bottles to protect them from light degradation. Always label preparations with the date made and the expected shelf life to ensure they are used within a period when they are most potent.

Monitoring and Adjusting Based on Response

Observing and adjusting based on the individual's response to a remedy is a cornerstone of safe and effective herbal practice. What works well for one person may not be as effective for another, due to differences in metabolism, health status, and other factors. Begin with conservative dosages and closely monitor the effects. Be prepared to adjust the dosage or switch to a different herb if the desired outcomes are not achieved or if adverse reactions occur.

Engaging with Professional Guidance

Despite the wealth of information available, engaging with healthcare professionals, particularly those knowledgeable in both conventional and herbal medicine, can provide invaluable insights into the safe and effective use of herbal remedies. These professionals can offer tailored advice, taking into account the individual's health history, current medications, and specific health objectives, ensuring that the use of herbal remedies contributes positively to the individual's overall health strategy.

By adhering to these principles, individuals can navigate the complexities of herbal medicine with confidence, maximizing the benefits while minimizing risks. This careful, informed approach supports the ultimate goal of the holistic family home apothecary: to nurture health and well-being through the thoughtful integration of natural remedies into daily life.

Setting Up Your Home Apothecary

When setting up your home apothecary, the first step is to identify a dedicated space that will serve as your herbal sanctuary. This space doesn't have to be large; a small cabinet, shelf, or even a portion of your kitchen counter can suffice, as long as it is solely dedicated to storing your herbs and preparation tools. The key is to choose a location that is away from direct sunlight, moisture, and extreme temperature changes to preserve the potency and efficacy of your herbs. A cool, dry place is ideal, such as a pantry or a closet.

Once you have selected the perfect spot, the next step is to gather the essential tools you will need for preparing and storing your herbal remedies. These tools include glass jars with tight-fitting lids for storing dried herbs and tinctures, a mortar and pestle for grinding herbs, a digital scale for precise measurements, and cheesecloth or a fine mesh strainer for filtering tinctures and infusions. It's also beneficial to have a selection of amber glass bottles, which are essential for storing tinctures and herbal oils, as they protect the contents from light, which can degrade the active compounds in herbs.

Labeling is another critical aspect of setting up your home apothecary. Every jar, bottle, and container should be clearly labeled with the name of the herb, the date it was processed or purchased, and the expected shelf life. This practice not only helps in organizing your apothecary but also ensures the safety and effectiveness of your remedies. Waterproof, adhesive labels are ideal for this purpose, and a permanent marker should be used to prevent the ink from fading over time.

In addition to the physical setup, creating a reference system within your apothecary is invaluable. This can be a digital document, a notebook, or index cards that contain information about each herb's properties, uses, and any safety precautions. Having this information at your fingertips will not only save time but will also enhance your understanding and confidence in using herbal remedies effectively.

As your apothecary grows, you may find it beneficial to categorize your herbs and remedies. Organizing your space into sections such as "culinary herbs," "medicinal tinctures," and "topical preparations" can streamline the process of finding what you need and keeping track of your inventory. This categorization can extend to your reference system, making it easier to cross-reference herbs and their uses.

The foundation of a successful home apothecary is not just in the physical setup but also in the commitment to maintaining a clean, organized, and well-documented space. Regular checks for expired products, restocking essential herbs and supplies, and keeping abreast of new herbal knowledge and practices will ensure your apothecary remains a reliable resource for natural health and wellness for your family.

To further enhance the functionality of your home apothecary, consider incorporating a small garden or collection of potted herbs that can be grown indoors or in your backyard. This not only ensures a fresh supply of herbs but also deepens your connection to the plants you use for healing. Herbs such as basil, mint, rosemary, and thyme are not only culinary treasures but also possess medicinal properties, making them perfect candidates for your apothecary garden. Utilize high-quality, organic soil and ensure proper drainage to promote healthy growth. Regular pruning and harvesting encourage the plants to thrive and provide you with a continuous supply of fresh herbs.

When it comes to expanding your home apothecary, exploring local farmers' markets and herbal shops can be a delightful way to discover new herbs and gain insights from seasoned herbalists. Building relationships with local growers and suppliers can also lead to sourcing higher-quality, ethically harvested herbs. Additionally, attending workshops or joining herbalist groups in your community can enhance your knowledge and skills, providing a supportive network for sharing experiences and remedies.

For those interested in creating more complex herbal preparations, investing in additional equipment such as an herb dehydrator, an oil infuser, or a small still for distilling essential oils can be worthwhile. These tools allow for a broader range of herbal products to be made at home, from dried herbs for tea blends to homemade essential oils for aromatherapy and skincare products. Remember, the key to mastering these techniques lies in patience and practice, as well as a willingness to learn from mistakes and successes alike.

Documentation of your herbal creations and their effects is also crucial for a thriving apothecary. Keeping a detailed journal of recipes, dosages, and personal or family reactions to various remedies will help you refine your practice and tailor remedies to specific needs. This record-keeping will prove invaluable over time, creating a personalized compendium of herbal knowledge that can be passed down through generations.

Finally, integrating technology into your home apothecary can streamline the management of your herbal inventory and reference materials. Digital apps for organizing recipes, tracking inventory levels, and setting reminders for planting, harvesting, or restocking supplies can enhance efficiency and ensure your apothecary remains well-maintained. Additionally, online forums and databases provide a wealth of information on herbal medicine, offering access to the latest research, traditional recipes, and community support.

By embracing these practices, your home apothecary will not only serve as a source of natural remedies but also as a sanctuary for learning and personal growth. The journey of building and nurturing your apothecary is continuous, evolving with your expanding knowledge of herbal medicine and the changing needs of your family. Through this process, you cultivate not only health and wellness but also a deeper appreciation for the natural world and its abundant healing gifts.

Essential Tools and Ingredients

In the realm of creating a holistic family home apothecary, the selection of essential tools and ingredients forms the cornerstone of your practice. To ensure the efficacy and safety of your remedies, a meticulous approach to choosing and utilizing these components is paramount. This section delves into the specifics of these tools and ingredients, providing guidance to navigate your choices with confidence.

For the preparation of herbal remedies, a high-quality mortar and pestle made from porcelain or granite is indispensable. The material should be non-porous to prevent the absorption of oils and flavors from the herbs. When grinding dried herbs, a porcelain mortar and pestle offer the ideal texture for breaking down the plant material into a fine powder, which is crucial for making potent and homogeneous mixtures.

Measuring tools are another critical component. Digital scales, capable of measuring to the nearest gram or ounce, are essential for ensuring precise dosages in your preparations. For liquid measurements, glass measuring cups with clear markings in ounces, milliliters, and tablespoons provide accuracy for tinctures, syrups, and other liquid remedies. The use of glass over plastic is recommended to avoid potential contamination from plasticizers.

When it comes to ingredients, the quality of herbs cannot be overstated. Organic herbs are preferred to minimize exposure to pesticides and chemicals. When sourcing herbs, whether dried or fresh, look for suppliers who provide transparent information about their farming practices and herb provenance. For dried herbs, ensure they are vibrant in color and aroma, as these qualities are indicative of their potency. Fresh herbs should be sourced locally when possible, ensuring they are harvested at the peak of their medicinal properties.

Carrier oils, such as jojoba, almond, and coconut oil, are used in the preparation of herbal-infused oils and salves. Select cold-pressed, organic oils as they retain more of their natural therapeutic properties. Each oil has its own shelf life and therapeutic benefits, so choosing the right oil for your preparation is key. For example, coconut oil has antimicrobial properties and a long shelf life, making it suitable for topical preparations intended for skin health.

Alcohol is used in the creation of tinctures due to its ability to extract and preserve the active constituents of herbs. A high-proof grain alcohol is ideal, but for those preferring a non-alcoholic alternative, vegetable glycerin or apple cider vinegar can be used. Each solvent extracts different compounds from the herbs, so the choice of solvent should be aligned with the intended use of the tincture.

For storage, amber glass bottles and jars with airtight lids are necessary to protect the remedies from light and air, which can degrade their quality over time. Tincture bottles should come equipped with droppers for ease of dosage. Additionally, labeling materials, including waterproof labels and a permanent marker, are essential for marking each preparation with its name, date, and dosage instructions.

The process of selecting and preparing these tools and ingredients is not merely a matter of logistics but a reflection of the holistic philosophy underpinning your home apothecary. Each choice, from the selection of ethically sourced herbs to the preference for organic carrier oils, contributes to the sustainability and efficacy of your practice. By adhering to these guidelines, you equip yourself with the foundational elements necessary to create safe, effective, and personalized herbal remedies for your family's wellness.

Organizing Your Space

Maximizing the functionality and efficiency of your home apothecary space requires thoughtful organization and the strategic use of storage solutions. After selecting the ideal location and gathering your essential tools and ingredients, the next step involves organizing these components in a way that makes them easily accessible while preserving their quality.

For dried herbs, invest in a variety of glass jars with airtight seals. These jars should come in several sizes to accommodate different quantities of herbs. To ensure optimal preservation, store these jars in a cabinet or on shelves that are not exposed to direct sunlight. The interior space should maintain a consistent temperature, ideally between 60-70°F (15-21°C), with low humidity to prevent the herbs from becoming damp or moldy. Silica gel packets can be placed inside the jars to absorb any excess moisture, further protecting the herbs' potency.

Labeling each jar with the herb's name, harvest date, and expiration date is crucial for effective organization. Consider implementing a color-coding system for the labels, using different colors to categorize herbs by their primary use—such as culinary, medicinal, or topical. This system enables you to quickly locate the herb you need without having to search through each jar. Additionally, arranging the jars alphabetically or by category can save time and streamline the preparation process.

For tinctures, extracts, and oils, amber glass bottles with droppers or pumps are preferred. These should be stored in a cool, dark place to protect the active compounds from degradation. If your space allows, dedicate a specific shelf or cabinet section exclusively for these liquids, grouping them by type or purpose. Implementing a first-in, first-out rotation system ensures that older preparations are used before newer ones, minimizing waste.

The organization of tools is equally important. A drawer or container designated for smaller items like measuring spoons, pipettes, and funnels keeps them from being misplaced and readily available when needed. Larger equipment, such as mortar and pestles, scales, and strainers, can be stored on a sturdy shelf or in a cabinet. If space is limited, consider using wall-mounted racks or magnetic strips to hang lightweight tools, keeping them off countertops but within easy reach.

Creating an inventory list can further enhance the organization of your home apothecary. This list should include each herb, preparation, and tool, along with quantities and locations. Keeping this list updated and easily accessible—either in a digital format or as a physical document—allows for quick reference and helps in maintaining stock levels, planning for replenishments, and avoiding duplications.

For those incorporating fresh herbs from a garden or indoor plants, consider setting up a small processing area near your storage space. This area can be equipped with cutting boards, scissors, and trays for cleaning and preparing the herbs before drying or using them fresh. A dehydrator, if available, can be placed in this area for convenience.

Efficient space organization extends to the maintenance of a clean and orderly environment. Regular cleaning of shelves, jars, and tools prevents dust accumulation and potential contamination. It also provides an opportunity to inspect your herbs and preparations for signs of spoilage or pest infestation, ensuring that only the highest quality ingredients are used in your remedies.

By implementing these organizational strategies, your home apothecary becomes not only a place of healing and wellness but also a reflection of your commitment to a holistic and sustainable lifestyle. The organized space fosters a serene environment where the preparation of natural remedies is both a pleasure and a practice, deeply rooted in the ancient traditions of herbal medicine while adapted to the modern world.

Basic Herbal Preparations

In the realm of home apothecary, mastering the art of basic herbal preparations is a crucial skill that empowers you to create effective, natural remedies tailored to your family's health needs. The process begins with understanding the various forms of herbal preparations, each serving a unique purpose and offering different benefits. The first and perhaps most foundational preparation we'll explore is the **tincture**.

Tinctures are concentrated herbal extracts made by soaking herbs in alcohol or a vinegar-based solvent. This method extracts the active compounds from the herbs, resulting in a potent liquid that can be taken in small doses. To create a tincture, start by selecting a high-proof alcohol, such as vodka or brandy, for its preservation qualities and ability to extract a wide range of plant constituents. For those preferring a non-alcoholic base, apple cider vinegar or vegetable glycerin are effective alternatives, though they may not extract as wide a range of compounds.

The process involves filling a clean, dry jar about half to two-thirds full with dried herbs. If using fresh herbs, chop them finely to increase the surface area for extraction and fill the jar loosely to allow for expansion. Next, pour the alcohol or alternative solvent over the herbs until they are completely submerged, leaving about an inch of space at the top of the jar. Seal the jar tightly and label it with the date and contents. Store the jar in a cool, dark place, shaking it daily for at least four to six weeks. The longer it sits, the stronger your tincture will be. After the desired steeping time, strain the liquid through a fine mesh strainer or cheesecloth into another clean jar or bottles, squeezing out as much liquid as possible. Label the tincture with its name and the date of completion. Tinctures can be stored in a cool, dark place for several years.

Moving on to **infused oils**, these are created by soaking herbs in a carrier oil to extract their active ingredients, resulting in a versatile preparation that can be used for cooking, skincare, or as a base for salves and balms. To make an infused oil, choose a carrier oil like olive, coconut, or almond oil for its own health benefits and compatibility with the chosen herb. Place dried herbs in a clean jar, and pour the carrier oil over the herbs until they are fully submerged. Cover the jar and place it in a warm, sunny spot for about 4-6 weeks, shaking it occasionally. For a quicker method, you can gently heat the oil and herbs over low heat for a few hours, being careful not to overheat or fry the herbs. After the infusion period, strain the oil through a fine mesh strainer or cheesecloth into a clean bottle or jar, and label it with the herb and date. Infused oils should be stored in a cool, dark place and typically last for up to a year.

These basic preparations form the cornerstone of home apothecary, allowing for a wide range of natural remedies and personal care products to be crafted from the comfort of your own home. With these techniques, you can begin to explore the vast world of herbal medicine, creating tinctures and infused oils that cater specifically to your family's health needs and preferences.

Salves and balms are another essential preparation in the home apothecary, offering targeted relief for a variety of skin conditions, wounds, and muscle pains. To create a salve, start by infusing your chosen herbs in a carrier oil, following the method described for infused oils. Once your herbal oil is ready, the next step involves combining it with beeswax to create a semi-solid consistency. The general ratio is one part beeswax to four parts infused oil, but this can be adjusted depending on the desired thickness of the final product. Gently melt the beeswax in a double boiler, then slowly add the infused oil, stirring continuously. If desired, essential oils can be added at this stage for additional therapeutic benefits and fragrance. Pour the mixture into clean tins or jars and allow it to cool and solidify. Label each container with the contents and date. Salves are best stored in a cool, dark place and typically last for up to a year.

Herbal teas and decoctions represent a more traditional approach to herbal medicine, allowing for the direct ingestion of the herbs' beneficial properties. Herbal teas are made by steeping dried or fresh herbs in hot water, a method suitable for delicate parts of the plant like leaves, flowers, and thin stems. To prepare, boil water and pour it over the herbs, covering them to prevent the escape of volatile oils. Steep for 5 to 15 minutes, depending on the herb and desired strength. Decoctions are prepared by simmering tougher plant parts, such as roots, bark, and seeds, in water for a longer period, typically 20 minutes to several hours. This method extracts the deep-seated constituents of the plant material. After preparing, strain the liquid and enjoy as is or sweeten with honey if desired. Both teas and decoctions can be consumed immediately or stored in the refrigerator for a few days.

The creation of herbal vinegars offers a flavorful way to preserve and consume the healing properties of herbs. Begin by filling a clean jar with fresh herbs, then cover completely with apple cider vinegar, ensuring all plant material is submerged to prevent mold growth. Seal the jar with a plastic lid or place parchment paper under a metal lid to prevent corrosion from the vinegar. Store the jar in a cool, dark place, shaking it every few days. After 4-6 weeks, strain the vinegar into a clean bottle, label it with the herb and date, and use it in dressings, marinades, or as a daily health tonic.

Each of these basic herbal preparations—tinctures, infused oils, salves and balms, herbal teas and decoctions, and herbal vinegars—serves as a foundation for building a comprehensive home apothecary. By mastering these techniques, you can harness the natural healing power of herbs to care for your family's health in a holistic and personalized manner. The process of creating these remedies not only deepens your connection to the natural world but also empowers you to take an active role in your family's wellness journey.

Tinctures and Extracts

Continuing from the foundational practices of creating tinctures, a deeper dive into the methodology reveals the importance of ratio precision and timing in the extraction process. For a standard tincture, the herb-to-solvent ratio is critical and often follows a 1:5 (herb weight in ounces to solvent volume in fluid ounces) ratio for dried herbs and a 1:2 ratio for fresh herbs. This precision ensures that the solvent sufficiently extracts the active constituents without becoming overly diluted. When using high-proof alcohol, a 40-50% concentration is generally effective for a broad range of herbs, balancing the extraction of both water-soluble and alcohol-soluble compounds. For those utilizing apple cider vinegar or vegetable glycerin, understanding that these solvents may extract a different spectrum of constituents is key. Apple cider vinegar, rich in acetic acid, can pull out minerals and other water-soluble compounds, making it ideal for mineral-rich herbs. Vegetable glycerin, being sweeter and thicker, is suitable for creating palatable preparations, especially for children, but may not extract certain compounds as effectively as alcohol.

The maceration time, typically ranging from four to six weeks, allows for a thorough extraction of the herbs' medicinal properties. However, this period can vary depending on the herb and the desired strength of the tincture. Agitation of the jar daily serves to mix the contents, preventing clumping of the herb and ensuring a consistent extraction process. After the maceration period, the straining process involves not just separating the solid herb particles from the liquid but also pressing or squeezing the marc (the spent plant material) to extract as much liquid as possible. This step is crucial as some of the most potent compounds may be held within the marc. The final tincture should be stored in amber or dark-colored glass bottles to protect it from light, which can degrade the active constituents over time. Labeling with the herb name, date of completion, and concentration of alcohol or alternative solvent provides essential information for future use and ensures proper dosage.

The creation of extracts extends beyond tinctures to include glycerites and acetracts (vinegar extracts), each offering unique benefits and considerations. Glycerites, made with vegetable glycerin, require a different ratio, often 1:8 for dried herbs, due to glycerin's lower solvency power. The sweetness and viscosity of glycerites make them particularly appealing for children's remedies or those sensitive to alcohol. Acetracts, or vinegar extracts, are valued for their ability to extract minerals and are made with a similar ratio to alcohol tinctures. The choice of solvent impacts not only the extraction of constituents but also the shelf life, with alcohol tinctures lasting several years, while glycerites and acetracts have a shorter shelf life, typically one to two years.

In addition to these liquid preparations, the practice of creating powdered extracts offers a more concentrated form of herbal medicine. This process involves evaporating the solvent from a liquid extract, leaving behind a concentrated powder that can be reconstituted with water or added to capsules for easy consumption. The concentration process requires careful temperature control to preserve the integrity of the active compounds, often utilizing low-heat evaporation or freeze-drying techniques.

Each of these methods—tinctures, glycerites, acetracts, and powdered extracts—provides a versatile approach to harnessing the therapeutic properties of herbs. The choice of method depends on the intended use, the specific properties of the herb, and the needs of the individual taking the remedy. By understanding the nuances of each extraction technique, practitioners of home apothecary can create a wide array of preparations tailored to the specific health needs of their family, ensuring that the ancient practice of herbal medicine continues to thrive in modern times.

Salves and Balms

Continuing with the preparation of salves and balms, after combining the infused oil with beeswax and achieving the desired consistency, the addition of essential oils can significantly enhance the therapeutic properties of your final product. When selecting essential oils for your salve or balm, consider the specific benefits you aim to achieve. For instance, lavender essential oil is renowned for its calming and anti-inflammatory properties, making it an excellent choice for salves intended to soothe skin irritations or promote relaxation. Meanwhile, peppermint essential oil offers cooling effects and can help relieve muscle pain when incorporated into balms. It is crucial to add essential oils only after removing the mixture from heat to preserve their volatile compounds. Typically, a ratio of 5-10 drops of essential oil per ounce of salve mixture is recommended, but this can vary depending on the oil's potency and the intended use of the product.

Once the essential oils are thoroughly mixed into the beeswax and infused oil base, the next step involves pouring the liquid mixture into containers. Selection of containers is an important consideration in the creation of salves and balms. Metal tins or small glass jars are commonly used due to their durability and ease of transport. Ensure the containers are clean and dry before use to prevent contamination. Pouring the mixture should be done carefully to avoid air bubbles, filling each container to just below the rim for a clean finish.

As the salves and balms cool, they will begin to solidify. This process can take several hours, and it is advisable to let them sit undisturbed in a cool, dark place to ensure even hardening. Once solidified, the salves and balms are ready for labeling. Similar to other herbal preparations, labeling should include the product name, the date of creation, and a list of ingredients. This practice not only helps in identifying the contents but also ensures safe and informed usage.

Storage of salves and balms is another critical aspect to ensure their longevity and efficacy. Ideally, they should be stored in a cool, dark place away from direct sunlight and heat sources. Under optimal conditions, salves and balms can maintain their quality for up to a year. However, it is important to monitor for any changes in texture, color, or scent, which may indicate spoilage. If any signs of degradation are observed, the product should be discarded to avoid skin irritation or diminished effectiveness.

For those interested in customizing the therapeutic effects of their salves and balms further, experimenting with different combinations of herbs and essential oils can be rewarding. For example, combining comfrey and calendula infused oils can create a powerful healing salve for cuts and scrapes, while a balm made with arnica infused oil and eucalyptus essential oil can be particularly effective for relieving sore muscles. The possibilities are vast, and with practice, you can develop formulations that cater specifically to your family's needs.

In addition to the therapeutic benefits, crafting your own salves and balms offers the satisfaction of creating natural, chemical-free products that nurture the body and spirit. It embodies the holistic philosophy of home apothecary, where the preparation of remedies is as much about the process and intention as it is about the healing properties of the ingredients. Through this practice, you not only provide care for your family but also deepen your connection to the natural world, fostering a lifestyle that values sustainability, health, and wellness.

Herbal Teas and Decoctions

Herbal teas and decoctions stand as a cornerstone in the practice of home apothecary, offering a method to extract the therapeutic properties of herbs in a form that is both accessible and enjoyable. The preparation of herbal teas involves steeping dried or fresh herbs in hot water, a process known as infusion, which allows the water-soluble components of the herbs to be released. Decoctions, on the other hand, involve simmering tougher plant materials, such as roots, bark, and seeds, in boiling water over a longer period, thereby extracting the deeper, water-soluble constituents that an infusion might not fully capture.

For the preparation of an herbal tea, begin by selecting a high-quality, non-reactive vessel, such as a ceramic or glass teapot. Measure approximately one teaspoon of dried herbs or one tablespoon of fresh herbs per cup of water, adjusting according to personal taste and the potency of the herb. Boil water and allow it to cool slightly before pouring over the herbs to avoid destroying delicate compounds through excessive heat. Cover the teapot or cup to prevent the escape of volatile oils and steep for 5 to 15 minutes, depending on the desired strength. Strain the tea to remove the plant material, and it is ready to be enjoyed. Sweeteners or lemon may be added according to personal preference, but often the natural flavors of the herbs are sufficient.

Creating a decoction requires a more prolonged process. Begin with cold water in a pot, adding about one teaspoon of dried, coarsely ground herbs per cup of water. Slowly bring the mixture to a boil, then reduce the heat and simmer gently, covered, for 20 to 45 minutes. The length of time will depend on the specific herbs used and the desired strength of the decoction. It is important to keep the pot covered to ensure that the volatile oils are not lost to evaporation. Once the decoction is ready, strain the liquid from the plant material. Decoctions are typically stronger in flavor and may be diluted with additional water or mixed with herbal teas to improve taste.

The choice between making an herbal tea and a decoction depends largely on the part of the plant being used and the desired constituents to be extracted. Leaves and flowers are best suited to teas, while roots, bark, and seeds are more effectively processed into decoctions. However, some herbs can be prepared either way, with the method selected based on personal preference or specific health goals.

For those new to herbal preparations, starting with familiar herbs such as chamomile for relaxation, peppermint for digestion, or ginger for immune support can be a comforting introduction. It is essential to source herbs from reputable suppliers to ensure they are free from contaminants and have been properly identified. Additionally, understanding the properties and potential interactions of herbs is crucial, especially for those with existing health conditions or taking medication.

Incorporating herbal teas and decoctions into daily routines offers a simple yet profound way to connect with the healing power of plants. Whether seeking to calm the mind before sleep, support digestion, or fortify the body's defenses, these preparations provide a direct link to the natural world and its abundance of wellness-promoting resources. By mastering the art of tea and decoction making, individuals empower themselves and their families to harness the therapeutic benefits of herbs in a manner that is both ancient and profoundly relevant to contemporary life.

Chapter 2: Herbal Remedies for Everyday Ailments

Herbal remedies have been a cornerstone of family health care for centuries, offering natural, effective solutions for a wide range of everyday ailments. In this chapter, we delve into the preparation and use of herbal remedies for digestive health, a common concern among families. Digestive issues can range from mild discomfort, such as indigestion and bloating, to more severe conditions like irritable bowel syndrome (IBS) and gastroesophageal reflux disease (GERD). Fortunately, the world of herbal medicine provides a plethora of options to address these concerns gently and effectively.

Soothing Teas for Indigestion: One of the most accessible and immediate remedies for digestive discomfort is herbal tea. Peppermint tea, for example, is renowned for its ability to relax the digestive tract muscles, thereby easing indigestion. To prepare, steep 1-2 teaspoons of dried peppermint leaves in a cup of boiling water for 10 minutes. Strain and enjoy the tea warm, ideally between meals to maximize its digestive benefits. Similarly, ginger tea can be made by simmering a 1-inch piece of fresh ginger root in 2 cups of water for 10 minutes. Ginger's anti-inflammatory and anti-nausea properties make it a versatile remedy for a variety of digestive issues, including morning sickness.

Natural Probiotics and Prebiotics: The health of our gut microbiome plays a crucial role in overall digestive health. Incorporating natural sources of probiotics and prebiotics into the diet can significantly improve gut flora balance. Fermented foods like sauerkraut, kimchi, and kefir are rich in probiotics, the beneficial bacteria that support gut health. To prepare homemade sauerkraut, thinly slice a head of cabbage and massage it with about 1.5 tablespoons of sea salt until it releases its juice. Pack the cabbage tightly into a clean jar, ensuring the liquid covers it completely, and let it ferment at room temperature for 3 to 10 days. Prebiotics, on the other hand, serve as food for these beneficial bacteria. Foods high in dietary fiber, such as garlic, onions, and bananas, are excellent prebiotic sources that can be easily incorporated into daily meals.

Immune Support: Elderberry syrup is a potent herbal remedy for boosting the immune system, especially during cold and flu season. Rich in antioxidants and vitamins, elderberry can help reduce the duration and severity of respiratory infections. To make elderberry syrup at home, combine 1/2 cup of dried elderberries with 3 cups of water and bring to a boil. Reduce heat and simmer until the liquid is reduced by half, about 45 minutes. Strain the mixture, pressing the berries to extract all the liquid. While still warm, add 1 cup of honey, stirring until fully dissolved. Store the syrup in a clean, airtight bottle in the refrigerator. Adults can take 1 tablespoon daily for immune support, and children over the age of one can take 1 teaspoon daily.

Herbal Antivirals: In addition to elderberry, several other herbs possess strong antiviral properties that can be beneficial in preventing and fighting viral infections. Echinacea, for example, is widely used to enhance the immune response. A simple echinacea tea can be made by steeping 1 teaspoon of dried echinacea root or leaves in a cup of boiling water for 15 minutes. For best results, begin consuming echinacea tea at the first sign of illness and continue for up to a week to support the immune system.

As we explore these remedies, it's important to remember that while herbal treatments can offer significant benefits, they should be used with care and respect for their potency. Always consult with a healthcare professional before starting any new herbal regimen, especially for those with pre-existing conditions or who are pregnant or breastfeeding. Additionally, sourcing high-quality, organic herbs is crucial to ensure the safety and efficacy of these remedies. By integrating these natural solutions into our wellness routines, we can harness the power of plants to support and enhance our family's health.

Stress and Sleep: Lavender is a well-known herb for reducing stress and promoting sleep. A simple lavender tea can be made by steeping 1 teaspoon of dried lavender flowers in a cup of boiling water for 7 minutes. This calming tea is best enjoyed in the evening to prepare the body and mind for restful sleep. Additionally, creating a sleep-promoting tincture involves combining valerian root, another herb recognized for its sedative properties, with a solvent like high-proof alcohol. Use a ratio of 1:5, with 1 part of dried valerian root to 5 parts of alcohol, and let the mixture sit for a month, shaking it daily. Straining the mixture yields a potent tincture, of which 1-2 teaspoons can be taken before bedtime to aid sleep.

Relaxing Herbal Baths: Incorporating herbs into a warm bath can provide a deeply relaxing experience, aiding in stress relief and promoting better sleep. A soothing bath can be prepared by filling a muslin bag with calming herbs such as chamomile, lavender, and rose petals. Secure the bag and let it steep in the bathwater as it fills, releasing the therapeutic properties of the herbs. For an enhanced experience, essential oils from these herbs can also be added to the bathwater, providing aromatherapy benefits that further relax the mind and body.

Sleep-promoting Tinctures: In addition to the valerian root tincture mentioned earlier, a tincture combining hops and passionflower can also support better sleep. These herbs work synergistically to calm the nervous system and improve sleep quality. To create this tincture, use a 1:5 ratio of dried hops and passionflower to alcohol, allowing the mixture to macerate for four weeks. This tincture can be taken in the evening, with dosages ranging from 1-2 teaspoons, to facilitate a restful night's sleep.

Natural Pain Relief: Willow bark has been used for centuries as a natural remedy for pain and inflammation. Its active component, salicin, is similar to the active ingredient in aspirin. A tea made from willow bark can be prepared by simmering 1-2 teaspoons of the dried bark in 2 cups of water for 10-15 minutes. This tea can be consumed up to twice daily for relief from headaches, muscle pain, and other inflammatory conditions. Additionally, turmeric, with its potent anti-inflammatory compound curcumin, can be incorporated into daily meals or taken as a supplement to support pain relief.

Anti-inflammatory Herbs: Ginger and turmeric are powerful anti-inflammatory herbs that can be easily included in the diet to combat inflammation. A daily anti-inflammatory tea can be made by simmering freshly grated ginger and turmeric root in water for 10-15 minutes. Adding a pinch of black pepper increases the absorption of curcumin from turmeric. This tea not only helps reduce inflammation but also boosts the immune system.

Herbal Poultices for Pain: Creating a poultice with herbs such as arnica, comfrey, or St. John's wort can provide localized relief for pain and swelling. To make a poultice, grind the chosen herb to a paste, mixing it with a small amount of warm water if necessary. Apply the paste directly to the affected area, covering it with a clean cloth or gauze, and secure it in place. The poultice can be left on for several hours or overnight, providing soothing relief and aiding in the healing process.

By incorporating these herbal remedies and preparations into our daily routines, we empower ourselves and our families with natural, effective solutions for managing stress, sleep, and pain. These practices not only foster physical well-being but also deepen our connection to the natural world, supporting a holistic approach to health that benefits both our bodies and the environment.

Digestive Health

To further support digestive health, **Fennel Seed Tea** emerges as a traditional remedy, particularly beneficial for alleviating gas and bloating. To prepare, crush 1 teaspoon of fennel seeds to release their volatile oils, which are responsible for their digestive benefits. Boil 1 cup of water and pour it over the crushed seeds, allowing it to steep for 8 to 10 minutes. This tea can be consumed after meals to aid digestion and provide relief from discomfort.

Licorice Root is another herb with profound benefits for the digestive system, especially in managing conditions like acid reflux and stomach ulcers. For a soothing licorice root tea, add 1 teaspoon of dried licorice root to a cup of boiling water. Steep for 10 to 15 minutes. Due to its sweet flavor, additional sweeteners are usually not necessary. However, it is important to note that licorice root should be used cautiously, particularly by those with high blood pressure, and should not be consumed in large quantities or for extended periods.

Incorporating **Aloe Vera Juice** into the diet can also support digestive health by soothing the lining of the stomach and intestines, promoting regularity, and aiding in the healing of digestive tracts. For optimal benefits, look for pure aloe vera juice that is free from aloin, which can be a potent laxative and may cause discomfort for some individuals. A recommended starting dose is 2 to 4 ounces of juice per day, which can be taken directly or diluted in water or another juice. Always start with a small dose to assess tolerance.

Apple Cider Vinegar (ACV) has been touted for its potential to improve digestion, primarily by increasing stomach acidity which can aid in the digestion of food and absorption of nutrients. To utilize ACV, mix 1 tablespoon with a glass of water and consume before meals. This remedy is particularly beneficial for those who suspect they have low stomach acid. However, due to its acidity, it's advisable to start with a lower dose to ensure it agrees with your system and to prevent potential enamel erosion over time.

Digestive Bitters are a blend of bitter herbs that can be taken before meals to stimulate digestive juices, improve bile flow, and support overall digestion. Common ingredients in digestive bitters include dandelion, gentian root, and burdock root. To use, add a few drops of a commercial digestive bitters preparation to water and drink it 15 to 30 minutes before eating. This ancient remedy supports the body's natural digestive processes and can be particularly helpful when indulging in a larger or richer meal than usual.

Probiotic-Rich Foods play a crucial role in maintaining a healthy gut microbiome, which is essential for optimal digestion and overall health. Incorporating foods like yogurt, kefir, and fermented vegetables into your diet can help increase the diversity and abundance of beneficial gut bacteria. When selecting yogurt or kefir, opt for products that list "live and active cultures" on the label to ensure you're getting a good source of probiotics. For those making fermented vegetables at home, ensure a clean environment to avoid contamination and allow for proper fermentation to occur.

By integrating these natural remedies and practices into your daily routine, you can support and enhance your digestive health, contributing to a foundation of overall wellness for you and your family. Remember, while these remedies can offer significant benefits, it's important to listen to your body and consult with a healthcare professional if you have any concerns or pre-existing conditions.

Soothing Teas for Indigestion

Chamomile tea emerges as a gentle, yet powerful, herbal remedy for soothing indigestion and calming an upset stomach. To harness the full potential of chamomile, it's advisable to use 1-2 teaspoons of dried chamomile flowers per cup of boiling water. The preparation involves pouring the boiling water over the chamomile flowers and allowing the mixture to steep for 5 to 10 minutes. This steeping time ensures the extraction of the chamomile's beneficial compounds, such as bisabolol, which is known for its anti-inflammatory and antispasmodic properties. Straining the tea into a cup, one can enjoy this soothing beverage up to three times a day, especially after meals or before bedtime, to facilitate digestion and promote relaxation.

For those experiencing more severe digestive discomfort or bloating, adding a slice of fresh ginger to the chamomile tea can enhance its digestive benefits. Ginger, with its well-documented gastroprotective effects, can help to increase gastric motility, thereby relieving discomfort associated with indigestion. The combination of chamomile and ginger not only amplifies the tea's soothing effects but also adds a warm, comforting flavor profile that many find pleasant.

In the case of persistent indigestion, incorporating lemon balm into the herbal tea blend offers additional relief. Lemon balm, recognized for its calming effects on the digestive system, can be added by using 1 teaspoon of dried lemon balm leaves per cup of boiling water. When combined with chamomile, the lemon balm enhances the tea's overall efficacy in combating indigestion, thanks to its antiviral and antispasmodic properties. This blend is particularly beneficial in the evening, as lemon balm also contributes to a sense of calm and can aid in achieving a restful night's sleep.

For individuals seeking a remedy that also supports liver function, milk thistle tea can be a valuable addition to the digestive health regimen. Milk thistle, known for its hepatoprotective qualities, aids in the regeneration of liver cells and supports the liver in its role of detoxification. Preparing milk thistle tea involves steeping 1 teaspoon of crushed milk thistle seeds in a cup of boiling water for 15 to 20 minutes. This longer steeping time is necessary to extract the silymarin, the active compound in milk thistle that is responsible for its therapeutic effects. Consuming milk thistle tea once daily can contribute to improved digestion and overall liver health.

Lastly, for those who prefer a milder tea, fennel tea serves as an excellent choice for easing indigestion and reducing gas. Fennel seeds contain compounds that relax the smooth muscles of the gastrointestinal system, thereby alleviating bloating and gas pains. To prepare fennel tea, crush 1 teaspoon of fennel seeds to release their essential oils, then steep in a cup of boiling water for 8 to 10 minutes. This tea can be enjoyed after meals to aid in digestion and provide a refreshing, slightly sweet taste.

By selecting and preparing these teas with care, individuals can effectively manage indigestion and promote digestive health naturally. It's important to source high-quality, organic herbs to ensure the purity and potency of the teas. Additionally, while these herbal teas offer significant benefits, it's crucial to monitor one's response and consult with a healthcare professional if symptoms persist, as they may be indicative of a more serious underlying condition. Through the thoughtful integration of these herbal teas into one's daily routine, it's possible to support and enhance digestive wellness, contributing to an overall sense of well-being and vitality.

Natural Probiotics and Prebiotics

Incorporating natural probiotics and prebiotics into one's diet is a foundational step towards enhancing digestive health, a vital component of overall wellness. Probiotics, the live beneficial bacteria that inhabit the gut, play a critical role in digestion, immune function, and even mental health. Prebiotics, on the other hand, are non-digestible fibers that serve as food for these probiotic bacteria, encouraging their growth and activity. Understanding how to effectively integrate these elements into daily nutrition can significantly impact one's health positively.

To begin with probiotics, fermented foods stand out as the most potent and natural sources. Beyond the commonly known sauerkraut, kimchi, and kefir, incorporating a variety of fermented foods ensures a broad spectrum of probiotic strains. For instance, traditional Japanese miso, made from fermented soybeans, rice, or barley, offers a unique blend of bacteria and enzymes beneficial for the gut. When preparing miso soup, it's crucial to add the miso paste to the broth at the end of cooking, ensuring the water is not boiling. This preserves the live cultures and maximizes the probiotic benefits. Similarly, tempeh, a fermented soy product, can be marinated and cooked to serve as a probiotic-rich protein source in meals.

Turning to prebiotics, incorporating a diverse range of high-fiber foods into the diet is key. Artichokes, chicory root, and dandelion greens are excellent sources of inulin, a type of soluble fiber that promotes the growth of healthy gut bacteria. These can be integrated into the diet by adding artichokes to salads, using chicory root as a coffee substitute, or sautéing dandelion greens as a side dish. Additionally, whole grains such as barley and oats are rich in beta-glucan, a prebiotic fiber that supports immune health and enhances the growth of beneficial gut bacteria. Incorporating these grains into breakfast cereals, soups, and bread can significantly contribute to one's prebiotic intake.

Moreover, the preparation and consumption of these foods require careful consideration to preserve their probiotic and prebiotic benefits. For example, overcooking high-fiber vegetables can break down their prebiotic fibers, reducing their effectiveness. Thus, lightly steaming or eating them raw when possible is advisable. When it comes to probiotic foods, storage is also crucial. Fermented foods should be stored in the refrigerator to maintain the viability of the probiotic cultures. Ensuring that these foods are consumed before their expiration date is essential to receive their full health benefits.

In addition to dietary sources, supplementation can also play a role in enhancing one's probiotic and prebiotic intake. However, selecting high-quality supplements is paramount. For probiotics, choosing supplements that guarantee live and active cultures through the end of shelf life is crucial. For prebiotics, opting for supplements that specify the type and amount of prebiotic fibers, such as FOS (fructooligosaccharides) or GOS (galactooligosaccharides), can offer targeted support for digestive health.

Lastly, it's important to gradually introduce probiotics and prebiotics into the diet, especially for individuals new to these foods or with sensitive digestive systems. Starting with small servings and slowly increasing the amount can help the gut microbiome adjust without causing discomfort. Monitoring one's response to these dietary changes is also important, as individual tolerances can vary. Through mindful incorporation of natural probiotics and prebiotics, individuals can nurture their gut microbiome, laying a strong foundation for digestive health and overall wellness.

Immune Support

To bolster the immune system naturally, it's essential to incorporate **Astragalus Root** into your wellness regimen. This adaptogenic herb has been revered in traditional Chinese medicine for centuries, known for its ability to enhance the body's resistance to infections. To harness its benefits, start by acquiring dried astragalus root from a reputable source, ensuring it's organic to avoid contaminants. Prepare a decoction by simmering 1 to 2 tablespoons of sliced astragalus root in 2 cups of water for approximately 30 to 45 minutes. This slow cooking process extracts the root's immune-stimulating polysaccharides. Strain and consume the decoction once daily, ideally in the morning to kickstart your immune defenses. For a more convenient approach, astragalus is also available in capsule or tincture form, with dosage recommendations provided by the manufacturer.

Vitamin D, often referred to as the sunshine vitamin, plays a pivotal role in immune function. While sunlight exposure is the most natural way to obtain vitamin D, geographic location and lifestyle can limit sun exposure. Consider supplementing with vitamin D3, aiming for 1,000 to 2,000 IU daily, based on your healthcare provider's advice. Select a supplement that includes vitamin K2, which aids in the proper absorption and utilization of vitamin D.

Incorporating **Zinc** into your diet is another effective strategy for immune support. This trace mineral is crucial for the development and function of immune cells. To ensure adequate zinc intake, focus on foods rich in zinc such as pumpkin seeds, cashews, chickpeas, and spinach. For those considering zinc supplements, a daily dose of 8 to 11 mg for adults is generally recommended, but it's crucial not to exceed the upper limit of 40 mg per day to avoid adverse effects.

Probiotics are beneficial bacteria that support not only gut health but also the immune system. Incorporate probiotic-rich foods like yogurt, kefir, sauerkraut, and kimchi into your diet. For those preferring supplements, choose a probiotic with at least 1 billion CFUs and a variety of strains, including Lactobacillus and Bifidobacterium, taking it according to the product's instructions.

Elderberry is well-known for its immune-boosting properties, particularly in fighting viral infections. To make elderberry syrup, simmer 1 cup of dried elderberries in 4 cups of water for 45 minutes, then strain. Add 1 cup of honey to the strained liquid, mixing thoroughly. Store this syrup in a glass bottle in the refrigerator and consume 1 tablespoon daily for immune support. Elderberry supplements are also an option, with dosage following the manufacturer's guidelines.

Garlic, with its potent antiviral and antibacterial properties, is a powerful ally for the immune system. Incorporate fresh garlic into your meals, aiming for 1 to 2 cloves per day. For those who prefer not to consume fresh garlic, aged garlic supplements are an effective alternative, with suggested dosages provided on the product label.

Green Tea is rich in antioxidants, particularly epigallocatechin gallate (EGCG), which enhances immune function. Aim to drink 2 to 3 cups of green tea daily. Choose organic green tea leaves or bags to avoid pesticides and maximize health benefits.

Regular Exercise is crucial for maintaining a robust immune system. Engage in at least 150 minutes of moderate aerobic exercise or 75 minutes of vigorous exercise each week, complemented by two sessions of muscle-strengthening activities. Exercise promotes circulation, allowing immune cells to move more efficiently throughout the body.

Adequate Sleep cannot be overstated in its importance for immune health. Adults should aim for 7 to 9 hours of quality sleep per night. Establish a regular sleep schedule, limit exposure to blue light from screens before bedtime, and create a restful environment to support sleep quality.

Stress Management plays a significant role in immune function. Chronic stress can suppress immune response, so incorporating stress-reduction techniques such as meditation, deep breathing exercises, or yoga into your daily routine is beneficial.

By integrating these natural remedies and lifestyle practices into your daily life, you can effectively support and enhance your immune system, providing a solid foundation for health and well-being.

Elderberry Syrup for Immune Boosting

The preparation of elderberry syrup as an immune booster involves a meticulous process that ensures the preservation of its medicinal properties. Elderberries, recognized for their antiviral and immune-enhancing capabilities, must be sourced with care. Opt for organically grown elderberries to avoid pesticide residues, which can undermine the syrup's health benefits. Begin by measuring one cup of dried elderberries, ensuring that they are free from any stems or unripe berries, which can contain harmful compounds.

To extract the elderberries' active components, combine them with four cups of filtered water in a heavy-bottomed saucepan. This ratio ensures a potent concentration of elderberry extract. Bring the mixture to a boil over medium heat, then reduce the heat to simmer. Cover the saucepan with a lid slightly ajar to allow steam to escape, which concentrates the syrup by reducing the liquid volume. Simmer the mixture for approximately 45 minutes, or until the liquid has reduced by half. This slow simmering process is crucial for extracting the elderberries' beneficial compounds without destroying their delicate phytochemicals.

After simmering, remove the saucepan from heat and allow the mixture to cool to a manageable temperature. Strain the liquid through a fine mesh strainer or cheesecloth into a large bowl, pressing on the elderberries to extract as much liquid as possible. Discard the used elderberries in an environmentally responsible manner, such as composting, to minimize waste.

To enhance the syrup's immune-boosting properties and shelf life, stir in one cup of raw, local honey to the strained elderberry liquid. Honey, a natural preservative and sweetener, also adds its own antibacterial and antiviral properties to the syrup. Ensure the mixture has cooled to below 104°F before adding honey to preserve its enzymes and nutrients. Mix thoroughly until the honey is completely dissolved.

Pour the finished elderberry syrup into sterilized glass bottles or jars. Label each container with the date of preparation to keep track of its freshness. Store the syrup in the refrigerator, where it will keep for several months due to the natural preservative qualities of honey. For daily immune support, adults can consume one tablespoon of elderberry syrup daily, while children over the age of one may take one teaspoon daily. During periods of increased risk, such as cold and flu season, the dosage can be safely doubled.

It's important to note that while elderberry syrup is a powerful tool for immune support, it should be part of a holistic approach to health that includes a balanced diet, regular exercise, adequate sleep, and stress management. Individuals with autoimmune conditions or those taking immunosuppressive medication should consult with a healthcare provider before incorporating elderberry syrup into their wellness routine, to avoid potential interactions. By following these detailed steps, you can create a potent and natural remedy that supports the body's defense mechanisms, contributes to overall health, and empowers you and your family with a proactive approach to wellness.

Herbal Antivirals

Continuing with the theme of bolstering the immune system through natural means, another potent herbal antiviral to consider is **Olive Leaf Extract**. Olive leaf, derived from the leaves of the olive tree (Olea europaea), has been used for centuries in traditional medicine to treat a variety of ailments. Its antiviral properties are primarily attributed to a compound called oleuropein, which has been shown to inhibit the replication of viruses by interfering with their protein production. To incorporate olive leaf extract into your wellness regimen, look for supplements in capsule or liquid extract form. The recommended dosage for adults is generally 500 to 1000 mg daily, taken with meals to enhance absorption. It's crucial to choose a product standardized to contain a specific percentage of oleuropein to ensure potency.

Lemon Balm (Melissa officinalis) is another herb celebrated for its antiviral effects, particularly against the herpes simplex virus, which causes cold sores. Lemon balm can be used topically in a cream or taken internally as a tea or tincture. To prepare lemon balm tea, steep 1 to 2 teaspoons of dried lemon balm leaves in boiling water for 10 to 15 minutes. This soothing tea can be consumed 2 to 3 times daily. For topical use, apply lemon balm cream to the affected area 3 to 4 times per day at the first sign of a cold sore. When selecting lemon balm products, ensure they are sourced from reputable suppliers and contain a high concentration of the active constituents.

Andrographis (Andrographis paniculata), often referred to as "Indian Echinacea," is another herb with significant antiviral properties. It's widely used in Ayurvedic medicine and has been studied for its effectiveness in reducing the severity and duration of upper respiratory infections. Andrographis supplements are available in tablet or capsule form. The standard dose for immune support is 400 mg of andrographis extract, taken twice daily with meals. It's important to start taking andrographis at the first sign of cold or flu symptoms for the best results. As with all supplements, selecting a high-quality product from a reputable manufacturer is essential.

In addition to these herbs, maintaining a healthy lifestyle that includes a balanced diet rich in fruits, vegetables, and whole grains, regular physical activity, adequate hydration, and stress management techniques is vital for supporting the body's natural defense mechanisms. Incorporating herbal antivirals can provide an extra layer of protection against pathogens, but they should complement, not replace, foundational health practices.

When introducing any new supplement into your routine, especially herbal antivirals, it's advisable to consult with a healthcare professional, particularly if you have underlying health conditions or are taking prescription medications. This ensures that the supplements will not interact negatively with existing treatments and are appropriate for your health needs. Monitoring your body's response to these natural remedies is also important, as individual reactions can vary. By carefully selecting and using these herbal antivirals, you can enhance your immune system's ability to fend off viral infections, contributing to your overall health and well-being.

Stress and Sleep

For those seeking to alleviate stress and improve sleep through natural means, **Lavender** stands out as a remarkable herb with a long history of use for its calming and sedative properties. To incorporate lavender into your evening routine, consider preparing a lavender tea by steeping 1 to 2 teaspoons of dried lavender flowers in a cup of boiling water for 10 minutes. Strain the tea and drink it approximately 30 minutes before bedtime to help ease into a restful state. Additionally, lavender essential oil can be used in aromatherapy; add a few drops to a diffuser in your bedroom or dilute it with a carrier oil and apply to the temples or wrists before sleep.

Chamomile is another herb celebrated for its stress-reducing and sleep-promoting effects. Similar to lavender, chamomile tea can be made by infusing 1 to 2 teaspoons of dried chamomile flowers in boiling water for about 5 to 10 minutes. Drinking chamomile tea in the evening can help soothe the nervous system and promote a peaceful night's sleep. For those who prefer external applications, chamomile essential oil can be added to bathwater or used in a diffuser to create a calming atmosphere in the home.

Magnesium plays a critical role in the body's stress response and sleep regulation. Many people are unaware they are deficient in this vital mineral, which can exacerbate stress and disrupt sleep patterns. Incorporating magnesium-rich foods into your diet, such as spinach, almonds, and black beans, is one way to ensure adequate intake. Alternatively, a magnesium supplement taken 30 minutes before bedtime can help relax the muscles and nervous system, making it easier to fall asleep. Look for magnesium in forms that are easily absorbed by the body, such as magnesium glycinate or citrate, and start with a dose of 200 to 400 mg, based on your healthcare provider's recommendations.

Valerian Root has been used for centuries as a natural remedy to address insomnia and reduce anxiety. To benefit from valerian root's sleep-enhancing properties, consider taking a supplement 30 minutes to 2 hours before bedtime. The standard dosage for adults is between 300 to 600 mg. It's important to note that valerian root works best when used consistently over a period of time, rather than as a one-time solution. As with any supplement, consult with a healthcare professional before incorporating valerian root into your routine, especially if you are pregnant, nursing, or taking other medications.

Mindfulness and Meditation practices can significantly impact stress levels and improve sleep quality. Dedicate time each evening to unwind and practice mindfulness or meditation. This could involve guided meditation sessions, deep breathing exercises, or simply sitting quietly and focusing on the present moment. Establishing a regular mindfulness practice can help reduce overall stress levels and make it easier to fall asleep and stay asleep through the night.

Regular Physical Activity is essential for managing stress and promoting healthy sleep patterns. Engage in at least 30 minutes of moderate exercise most days of the week. Activities such as walking, cycling, or yoga can help reduce stress hormones and improve sleep quality. However, avoid vigorous exercise close to bedtime as it can energize the body and make it more difficult to fall asleep.

By incorporating these natural remedies and practices into your daily routine, you can create a holistic approach to managing stress and improving sleep. Remember, consistency is key, and it may take some time to notice significant changes. Always consult with a healthcare provider before starting any new supplement or drastically changing your diet or exercise regimen, especially if you have existing health conditions or concerns.

Relaxing Herbal Baths

For a deeply relaxing herbal bath that aids in stress relief and promotes better sleep, begin by selecting herbs known for their calming properties. **Epsom salt**, rich in magnesium, serves as the base for muscle relaxation, while **lavender** and **chamomile** provide soothing aromatherapy benefits. To create a more complex bath blend, consider adding **rose petals** for their gentle fragrance and **eucalyptus** for its respiratory benefits, especially useful before bedtime.

Materials Needed:

- 2 cups of Epsom salt
- 1/2 cup of baking soda (to soften the water and skin)
- 1/4 cup of dried lavender flowers
- 1/4 cup of dried chamomile flowers
- 1/4 cup of dried rose petals (optional)
- 10 drops of eucalyptus essential oil (optional)
- A large bowl for mixing
- A small muslin bag or a large tea infuser

Preparation Steps:

1. In a large bowl, mix the Epsom salt and baking soda thoroughly. These compounds will serve as the foundation of your herbal bath, providing both skin-softening and muscle-relaxing benefits.
2. Gently stir in the dried lavender flowers, chamomile flowers, and optional rose petals into the salt mixture. These herbs are chosen for their proven ability to reduce stress and promote relaxation.
3. Add the eucalyptus essential oil to the mixture, if using. This step is optional but recommended for its ability to enhance respiratory relaxation and contribute to overall stress relief.
4. Once all the ingredients are well combined, transfer the mixture to a muslin bag or large tea infuser. This will prevent the herbs from dispersing into the bath water, making cleanup easier and preventing any potential drain clogs.
5. To use, simply place the filled muslin bag or tea infuser under the faucet as you fill your bathtub with warm water. The pressure from the water will help release the essential oils and herbal properties, infusing your bath with a soothing blend.
6. For optimal relaxation, soak in the herbal bath for at least 20 minutes. This allows enough time for the magnesium from the Epsom salt to be absorbed through the skin, aiding in muscle relaxation, while the herbal aromas work to calm the mind.

Additional Tips:

- Ensure the water temperature is comfortably warm but not too hot, as excessive heat can exacerbate stress rather than alleviate it.
- Consider dimming the lights or using candles to create a serene atmosphere that encourages relaxation.
- Soft, instrumental music or nature sounds can further enhance the calming experience of your herbal bath.
- Stay hydrated by drinking a glass of water before and after your bath to replenish any fluids lost through sweating in the warm water.
- Practice deep breathing exercises while soaking in the bath to maximize stress relief and promote a state of mindfulness.

By incorporating these steps into your evening routine, you can create a tranquil spa experience in the comfort of your own home. This herbal bath blend not only aids in stress reduction and sleep improvement but also offers a moment of self-care that can be beneficial for both physical and mental well-being.

Sleep-Promoting Tinctures

In the realm of natural remedies for enhancing sleep quality, tinctures stand out for their potency and ease of use. A tincture is essentially a concentrated herbal extract made by soaking herbs in alcohol or vinegar, which acts as a solvent to extract the active compounds from the herbs. This section delves into the preparation of sleep-promoting tinctures, focusing on herbs known for their sedative properties, such as valerian root, passionflower, and hops.

To begin crafting a sleep-promoting tincture, select high-quality, dried herbs. Valerian root is renowned for its ability to improve sleep quality and ease falling asleep, passionflower contributes to reducing anxiety and insomnia, and hops, typically known for its use in brewing beer, also possesses sedative effects beneficial for sleep.

Materials Needed:
- Dried valerian root, passionflower, and hops (available at health food stores or online herbal suppliers)
- High-proof alcohol (at least 40% alcohol by volume, such as vodka or brandy) or apple cider vinegar for a non-alcoholic option
- A clean, dry glass jar with a tight-fitting lid
- A dark glass dropper bottle for storing the finished tincture
- Cheesecloth or a fine mesh strainer
- A small funnel

Preparation Steps:
1. Begin by measuring out approximately 1 part dried herbs to 4 parts alcohol or vinegar. This ratio ensures that the solvent is strong enough to extract the beneficial compounds from the herbs. If using a combination of herbs, maintain the overall ratio but divide the herbs equally according to weight.
2. Place the dried herbs in the glass jar and pour the alcohol or vinegar over them, making sure the herbs are completely submerged. If they float to the top, use a clean spoon to press them down and ensure they are fully covered by the solvent.
3. Seal the jar tightly and label it with the date and contents. Store the jar in a cool, dark place, such as a cupboard or pantry, away from direct sunlight. The darkness and stable temperature help preserve the tincture's potency.
4. Shake the jar gently every day to facilitate the extraction process. This action helps the solvent to more effectively break down the plant material and absorb the active compounds.

5. After 4 to 6 weeks, the tincture will be ready for straining. Open the jar and use cheesecloth or a fine mesh strainer to filter out the plant material, squeezing or pressing to extract as much liquid as possible.
6. Using a funnel, transfer the strained liquid into a dark glass dropper bottle. The dark glass helps protect the tincture from light, which can degrade its quality over time.
7. Label the dropper bottle with the tincture's name and the date of bottling. Stored properly, the tincture can last for several years.

Usage Guidelines:
- For sleep support, the recommended dosage of the tincture is typically 1 to 2 milliliters (about 20 to 40 drops), taken 30 minutes to an hour before bedtime. However, it's important to start with the lower end of this range and observe how your body responds, as sensitivity to herbal remedies can vary greatly among individuals.
- The tincture can be taken directly under the tongue for rapid absorption or diluted in a small amount of water or tea if preferred. Some find the taste of herbal tinctures to be strong or bitter, so dilution may make ingestion more palatable.

Considerations:
- Always consult with a healthcare provider before adding a new supplement to your routine, especially if you are pregnant, nursing, or taking prescription medications, as herbs can interact with some medications.
- Be patient with the effects of herbal tinctures. While some individuals may notice improvements in sleep quality relatively quickly, others may need to use the tincture consistently for a few weeks to experience the full benefits.

By integrating sleep-promoting tinctures into your evening routine, you can harness the power of herbs to support restful sleep naturally. This method of preparation allows for the creation of a potent, concentrated remedy that can be easily customized to suit individual needs and preferences, offering a practical and effective approach to enhancing sleep quality and overall well-being.

Chapter 3: Natural First Aid

For effective **natural pain relief**, understanding the properties and applications of **anti-inflammatory herbs** is crucial. These herbs, such as turmeric, ginger, and white willow bark, have been used for centuries to alleviate pain and reduce inflammation naturally. When incorporating these herbs into your home apothecary for pain management, precision in preparation and dosage is key to maximizing their benefits while ensuring safety.

Turmeric, known for its active compound **curcumin**, offers significant anti-inflammatory benefits. To harness turmeric's full potential, it can be used both internally and externally. For internal use, incorporating turmeric into your diet is beneficial, but for more concentrated effects, a turmeric supplement may be more effective. Look for supplements containing **piperine**, which enhances curcumin absorption, and start with a dosage of 500 mg twice daily, adjusting as necessary based on your response and healthcare provider's advice. For external application, creating a paste from turmeric powder and water and applying it to the affected area can help reduce inflammation and pain. Ensure the paste is thick enough to stay on the skin and cover it with a bandage if necessary to keep it in place.

Ginger, another powerful anti-inflammatory herb, can be used in various forms, including fresh, dried, or as an extract. For pain relief, ginger tea is a simple and effective method. Slice or grate fresh ginger and steep it in boiling water for 10-15 minutes. Drinking two to three cups daily can help alleviate pain. Alternatively, ginger supplements can be taken, with a recommended dosage of 500 mg up to three times daily. Always start with the lower end of the dosage range and consult your healthcare provider, especially if you're taking blood thinners, as ginger can increase the risk of bleeding.

White Willow Bark, often referred to as nature's aspirin, contains **salicin**, a compound that the body converts into salicylic acid, providing pain relief and anti-inflammatory effects. White willow bark can be taken as a tea, tincture, or in capsule form. For tea, simmer 1 to 2 teaspoons of dried bark in 8 ounces of water for 10 to 15 minutes, and drink up to three cups daily. If opting for a tincture, the suggested dosage is 1 to 2 ml three times daily. Capsules are another convenient option, with dosages typically ranging from 240 to 320 mg daily. It's important to note that white willow bark should not be used by children or adolescents due to the risk of Reye's syndrome, a rare but serious condition.

Herbal Poultices for pain involve the external application of herbs directly to the skin over the affected area. To make a poultice, select an anti-inflammatory herb such as turmeric, ginger, or crushed garlic, mix it with a small amount of warm water to form a paste, and apply it to the skin. Cover the poultice with a clean cloth or gauze and leave it in place for up to an hour. For conditions like arthritis or muscle pain, this method can provide localized relief.

Safety Considerations are paramount when using herbs for pain relief. Always consult with a healthcare provider before starting any new herbal regimen, especially if you have existing health conditions or are taking other medications. Be aware of potential interactions and side effects, such as gastrointestinal issues or allergic reactions, and adjust usage accordingly.

By integrating these anti-inflammatory herbs into your natural first aid toolkit, you can address pain effectively and safely, leveraging the healing power of nature. Remember, the key to successful herbal pain management is starting with small doses, monitoring your body's response, and adjusting as needed under the guidance of a healthcare professional.

Herbal Wound Care

For effective herbal wound care, it's essential to understand the properties of various herbs and how to apply them to cuts, scrapes, and bruises to promote healing and prevent infection. The following herbs have been recognized for their wound-healing properties: **Calendula**, **Comfrey**, **Plantain**, and **Tea Tree Oil**. Utilizing these herbs in your home apothecary can aid in the natural healing process.

Calendula (Calendula officinalis) is renowned for its anti-inflammatory, antimicrobial, and astringent properties. To prepare a calendula-infused oil, fill a jar with dried calendula flowers and cover them with a carrier oil such as olive or almond oil. Seal the jar and place it in a warm, sunny spot for 4 to 6 weeks, shaking it daily. Strain the oil using cheesecloth and store it in a dark glass bottle. Apply the oil directly to the wound or use it to make salves and creams.

Comfrey (Symphytum officinale) contains allantoin, a compound that promotes cell regeneration and can speed up the healing process. To make a comfrey poultice, grind fresh or dried comfrey leaves into a paste by mixing them with a small amount of hot water. Apply the paste directly to the affected area, cover it with a clean cloth, and secure it with a bandage. Leave it on for up to an hour before rinsing. Note: Comfrey should be used externally only and avoided on deep or puncture wounds.

Plantain (Plantago major) is a common weed that has powerful antiseptic and anti-inflammatory properties, making it ideal for wound care. To use, crush fresh plantain leaves with a mortar and pestle to release their juices. Apply the crushed leaves directly to the wound or mix them with a carrier oil to create a soothing balm.

Tea Tree Oil (Melaleuca alternifolia) is a potent antiseptic essential oil that can be applied to cuts and scrapes to prevent infection. Dilute tea tree oil with a carrier oil (10 drops of tea tree oil to 1 ounce of carrier oil) before applying to the skin to avoid irritation. Always perform a patch test on a small area of skin before using, as some individuals may be sensitive to tea tree oil.

Materials Needed:

- Dried calendula flowers
- Carrier oil (olive or almond oil)
- Clean, dry glass jar with a tight-fitting lid
- Cheesecloth
- Dark glass bottle for storage
- Fresh or dried comfrey leaves
- Hot water
- Clean cloth and bandage
- Fresh plantain leaves
- Mortar and pestle
- Tea tree essential oil

Preparation and Application Steps:

1. For calendula-infused oil, fill a jar with dried calendula flowers, cover with carrier oil, seal, and place in a warm spot for 4-6 weeks. Strain and store.
2. To make a comfrey poultice, grind comfrey leaves into a paste, apply to the wound, cover, and secure. Rinse after up to an hour.
3. Crush fresh plantain leaves and apply directly to the wound or mix with a carrier oil for a balm.
4. Dilute tea tree oil with a carrier oil before applying to the skin to prevent infection.

Safety Considerations:

- Always patch test herbal preparations to check for skin sensitivities.
- Consult with a healthcare provider before using herbal remedies, especially on deep or serious wounds.
- Use comfrey externally only and avoid applying to deep or puncture wounds.

By incorporating these herbs into your home apothecary for wound care, you can support the body's natural healing process while minimizing the risk of infection. Each herb offers unique properties beneficial for different types of wounds, allowing you to tailor your approach to the specific needs of each injury.

Antiseptic Sprays and Washes

Building on the foundation of herbal wound care, the creation of antiseptic sprays and washes is a critical step in preventing infection and promoting the healing of cuts, scrapes, and bruises. These solutions can be made from a variety of herbs known for their antimicrobial and healing properties, such as witch hazel, aloe vera, thyme, and eucalyptus. Each of these herbs brings unique benefits to the formulation, acting as powerful allies in the fight against bacteria and inflammation.

Witch hazel (Hamamelis virginiana) is a natural astringent, making it excellent for cleaning wounds and reducing swelling. To create a witch hazel antiseptic spray, begin by sourcing high-quality, alcohol-free witch hazel extract. Combine one part witch hazel extract with one part distilled water in a clean spray bottle. For added antimicrobial properties, include ten drops of tea tree essential oil for every 8 ounces of the mixture. Shake well before each use and spray directly onto the affected area, allowing it to air dry or gently patting it dry with a clean cloth.

Aloe vera, known for its soothing and healing properties, can be used to create a gentle wash for irritated skin or minor wounds. Extract the gel from an aloe vera leaf by slicing it open and scooping out the gel. Blend the gel with an equal part of distilled water to achieve a liquid consistency that can be easily applied. For an extra antimicrobial boost, add a few drops of lavender essential oil. This mixture can be stored in the refrigerator for up to one week. Apply it to the wound with a clean cotton ball or pad.

Thyme (Thymus vulgaris) and eucalyptus (Eucalyptus globulus) are potent antibacterial and antiseptic herbs, ideal for more robust antiseptic sprays. To harness their power, create a herbal infusion by boiling one tablespoon of dried thyme and one tablespoon of dried eucalyptus leaves in two cups of water for 15 minutes. Strain the herbs and allow the liquid to cool. Add this infusion to a spray bottle, combining it with an equal part of witch hazel. This spray can be used to disinfect wounds or as a general antiseptic spray for surfaces in your home apothecary.

Materials Needed:
- Alcohol-free witch hazel extract
- Distilled water
- Tea tree essential oil
- Aloe vera leaf
- Lavender essential oil
- Dried thyme leaves
- Dried eucalyptus leaves
- Clean spray bottles
- Cheesecloth or fine mesh strainer
- Clean cotton balls or pads

Preparation and Application Steps:
1. For the witch hazel antiseptic spray, mix one part witch hazel extract with one part distilled water in a spray bottle. Add ten drops of tea tree oil per 8 ounces of mixture.
2. To create the aloe vera wash, blend the gel from an aloe vera leaf with an equal part of distilled water. Add a few drops of lavender essential oil for its soothing and antimicrobial properties.
3. For the thyme and eucalyptus spray, boil one tablespoon each of dried thyme and eucalyptus in two cups of water for 15 minutes. Strain and cool the infusion before mixing with witch hazel in a spray bottle.
4. Apply the witch hazel spray directly to wounds, spraying from a distance and allowing to air dry. Use the aloe vera wash with a cotton ball or pad to gently clean the affected area. The thyme and eucalyptus spray can be used similarly or as a disinfectant for surfaces.

Safety Considerations:
- Perform a patch test with each new herbal preparation to ensure there is no allergic reaction.
- Consult with a healthcare provider before using these remedies on deep or serious wounds.
- Do not use essential oils undiluted directly on the skin to avoid irritation.
- Store homemade remedies in a cool, dark place and discard if there is any sign of spoilage or contamination.

By crafting your own antiseptic sprays and washes, you take an active role in the health and wellness of your family, utilizing the gifts of nature to protect and heal. These preparations, made from simple yet powerful ingredients, offer a natural alternative to commercial antiseptics, aligning with a holistic approach to health care and self-sufficiency.

Healing Salves for Cuts and Scrapes

Continuing from the foundation of herbal wound care, the creation of healing salves for cuts and scrapes represents a pivotal aspect of natural first aid, offering a protective barrier against infection while nurturing the skin's healing process. These salves combine the therapeutic properties of herbs with the soothing base of oils and beeswax, creating a potent remedy for minor wounds. To craft an effective healing salve, it is essential to select the right combination of herbs known for their wound-healing, anti-inflammatory, and antimicrobial properties, such as calendula, comfrey (for external use only), plantain, and tea tree oil.

The process begins with the infusion of selected herbs into a carrier oil. Olive oil is a popular choice due to its stability and skin-nourishing properties, but almond, coconut, or jojoba oil can also be used depending on skin sensitivities and preferences. To infuse the oil, combine 1 cup of carrier oil with ¼ cup of dried herbs of choice in a double boiler. Gently heat the mixture over low heat for 2 to 3 hours, ensuring the oil does not overheat or boil, to preserve the herbs' therapeutic properties. After the infusion process, strain the oil through cheesecloth to remove the herb particles, squeezing out as much oil as possible.

The next step involves the addition of beeswax, which solidifies the infused oil into a salve. For every cup of infused oil, approximately ¼ cup of beeswax pellets is needed. Adjust the amount of beeswax to achieve the desired consistency; more beeswax results in a firmer salve, while less produces a softer balm. Melt the beeswax in a double boiler, then slowly add the infused oil, stirring constantly until fully integrated. At this stage, essential oils can be added for additional therapeutic benefits and fragrance. Tea tree oil, known for its antiseptic properties, or lavender oil, for its soothing effect, are excellent choices. Use about 10-15 drops of essential oil per cup of salve mixture.

Once the mixture is homogeneous, carefully pour the liquid salve into clean, dry tins or glass jars. Allow the salve to cool and solidify at room temperature, avoiding the temptation to hasten the process in the refrigerator as this can cause condensation. Label each container with the ingredients and date of creation. Store the salve in a cool, dark place to maintain its potency.

When applying the salve to cuts and scrapes, ensure the wound has been properly cleaned and dried. Apply a small amount of salve to the affected area, then cover with a bandage if necessary. The natural ingredients not only help prevent infection but also soothe the skin and promote healing. It's important to monitor the wound for signs of infection or adverse reactions, especially when using new ingredients on sensitive skin.

Materials Needed:
- 1 cup of carrier oil (olive, almond, coconut, or jojoba oil)
- ¼ cup of dried herbs (calendula, comfrey for external use, plantain)
- ¼ cup of beeswax pellets (adjust for desired consistency)
- Cheesecloth
- Double boiler
- Clean, dry tins or glass jars for storage
- Essential oils (tea tree or lavender, optional)

Preparation and Application Steps:
1. Infuse carrier oil with dried herbs using a double boiler for 2 to 3 hours on low heat. Strain with cheesecloth.
2. Melt beeswax in a double boiler, then integrate the infused oil, stirring constantly.
3. Add essential oils if desired, mixing thoroughly.
4. Pour the mixture into containers, allowing it to solidify at room temperature.
5. Label containers with ingredients and date.
6. Apply to cleaned and dried wounds, covering with a bandage if necessary.

Safety Considerations:
- Always perform a patch test when using new ingredients to ensure no allergic reaction occurs.
- Consult with a healthcare provider before applying homemade salves to deep, puncture, or serious wounds.
- Be aware of the shelf life of your salve; homemade salves typically last for up to one year if stored properly.

By integrating these healing salves into your home apothecary, you empower yourself and your family with a natural, effective means of addressing minor wounds, embodying the principles of holistic health and self-care.

Natural Pain Relief

For those seeking **natural pain relief**, it's essential to understand the power of specific herbs and how to utilize them effectively. One of the most revered herbs for pain relief is **arnica (Arnica montana)**, widely recognized for its ability to reduce bruising and alleviate muscle soreness. To harness arnica's benefits, creating a simple **arnica oil infusion** is a practical method. Start by filling a jar halfway with dried arnica flowers, then cover the flowers completely with a carrier oil such as olive or almond oil. Seal the jar and place it in a warm, sunny spot for 4 to 6 weeks, shaking it every few days. After the infusion period, strain the oil through cheesecloth into a clean jar, and it's ready for use. Apply the oil directly to bruises or sore muscles, avoiding broken skin, as arnica is potent and should be used with caution.

Another remarkable herb for pain relief is **St. John's Wort (Hypericum perforatum)**, particularly effective for nerve pain. Similar to the arnica oil infusion, you can create a **St. John's Wort oil infusion** by soaking the dried herb in a carrier oil. This oil can then be applied to areas affected by nerve pain, such as the back or wrists. St. John's Wort is also known for its mood-lifting properties, providing a dual benefit for those experiencing pain-related stress or depression.

Capsaicin, derived from chili peppers, offers another avenue for pain relief, especially for joint and nerve pain. While capsaicin is available in over-the-counter creams, a homemade preparation can be made by mixing ground cayenne pepper with a carrier oil or unscented lotion. Start with a small amount of cayenne, as the heat can be intense, and apply it to a small test area before widespread use. Always wash hands thoroughly after application or consider using gloves during preparation to avoid irritation to the eyes or mucous membranes.

For those dealing with **headaches or migraines**, **peppermint oil** offers a cooling, soothing effect. A few drops of peppermint oil can be mixed with a carrier oil and massaged into the temples, forehead, and back of the neck. Peppermint's refreshing scent also helps to relieve the tension that often accompanies headaches.

Lastly, **ginger tea** serves as a gentle, internal remedy for inflammation and pain. Ginger contains compounds known as gingerols that have anti-inflammatory properties, making it an excellent choice for digestive discomfort, menstrual cramps, or muscle pain. To prepare, slice fresh ginger root and steep in boiling water for 10 to 15 minutes. The tea can be consumed two to three times a day for pain relief.

Materials Needed:
- Dried arnica flowers
- Dried St. John's Wort
- Carrier oil (olive, almond)
- Ground cayenne pepper or fresh chili peppers
- Peppermint essential oil
- Fresh ginger root
- Cheesecloth

- Clean jars for storage
- Unscented lotion (optional for capsaicin cream)

Preparation and Application Steps:
1. For arnica and St. John's Wort infusions, fill a jar halfway with the chosen dried herb and cover with carrier oil. Seal and place in a warm location for 4 to 6 weeks, shaking occasionally. Strain with cheesecloth before use.
2. To create a capsaicin cream, mix a small amount of ground cayenne with a carrier oil or unscented lotion and apply carefully to the affected area.
3. Mix peppermint oil with a carrier oil for headache relief and massage into the skin at pulse points.
4. For ginger tea, steep sliced ginger in boiling water, strain, and consume for internal pain relief.

Safety Considerations:
- Perform a patch test for topical preparations to ensure no allergic reaction occurs.
- Consult with a healthcare provider before using these remedies, especially if pregnant, nursing, or taking medication.
- Be cautious with the application of capsaicin; avoid contact with eyes and mucous membranes.
- Do not apply arnica to broken skin.

By incorporating these natural remedies into your pain management routine, you can leverage the healing properties of herbs and other natural ingredients to address various types of pain, from muscle soreness to nerve pain, in a holistic and effective manner.

Anti-inflammatory Herbs

Boswellia, also known as Indian Frankincense, emerges as a potent anti-inflammatory herb, particularly beneficial for those suffering from joint pain and conditions such as arthritis. The active components in Boswellia, known as boswellic acids, have been shown to inhibit the production of pro-inflammatory enzymes, offering relief without the side effects commonly associated with conventional pain medications. To incorporate Boswellia into a natural pain relief regimen, consider starting with a standardized extract of Boswellia serrata, aiming for a product that contains at least 60% boswellic acids. The recommended dosage typically ranges from 300 to 500 mg taken two to three times daily with food. It's important to note that while Boswellia supplements are widely available, quality can vary, so selecting a reputable brand that provides third-party testing is advisable to ensure purity and potency.

Another herb, Feverfew (Tanacetum parthenium), has a long history of use in traditional medicine for treating headaches, including migraines. The parthenolide compound, found in Feverfew, contributes to its anti-inflammatory and pain-relieving properties. For those looking to utilize Feverfew for headache relief, the herb can be consumed as a dried leaf capsule, liquid extract, or even as a tea. When choosing Feverfew supplements, opt for products labeled as "feverfew leaf" to ensure you're getting the herb in its most effective form. The typical dosage for preventing migraines is between 50 to 150 mg of dried Feverfew leaf daily, taken in divided doses. Though Feverfew is generally well-tolerated, it's advisable to start with a lower dose to assess tolerance.

In addition to these herbs, incorporating Omega-3 fatty acids into one's diet can further support the body's anti-inflammatory response. Found in high concentrations in fish oil, flaxseed, and walnuts, Omega-3s work by reducing the production of substances linked to inflammation. For those preferring a supplement form, fish oil capsules are an efficient way to increase Omega-3 intake, with a recommended dosage of 1,000 to 3,000 mg daily, depending on individual health goals and dietary restrictions.

When preparing herbal teas for pain relief, such as ginger or Feverfew tea, it's crucial to use purified water to avoid contaminants that could detract from the herbs' medicinal properties. Bring the water to a near boil, then pour over the herb, allowing it to steep for 10 to 15 minutes for maximum extraction of the active compounds. Straining the tea through a fine mesh strainer can remove particulates, providing a smooth tea experience.

For topical applications, such as creating a Boswellia or capsaicin cream, begin with a base of high-quality, unscented lotion or carrier oil like coconut or jojoba oil. Slowly incorporate the active ingredient, testing for desired consistency and potency. For capsaicin creams, a minute amount of ground cayenne pepper is mixed into the base. It's imperative to conduct a patch test on a small area of skin to ensure no adverse reaction occurs before widespread application.

Materials Needed:
- Standardized Boswellia extract (60% boswellic acids)
- Feverfew supplements (dried leaf capsule or liquid extract)
- Omega-3 supplements (fish oil capsules) or natural sources (flaxseed, walnuts)
- Purified water for herbal teas
- High-quality, unscented lotion or carrier oil for topical applications
- Fine mesh strainer for tea
- Ground cayenne pepper for capsaicin cream

Preparation and Application Steps:
1. For oral supplements like Boswellia and Feverfew, follow the recommended dosage on the product label, taking with food to enhance absorption.
2. To prepare herbal teas, steep the chosen herb in nearly boiling purified water for 10 to 15 minutes, strain, and consume as directed for pain relief.
3. For making topical creams, mix the active ingredient with the lotion or carrier oil until the desired consistency is reached, apply a small amount to a test area of skin before general use.

By carefully selecting and utilizing these anti-inflammatory herbs and supplements, individuals can address pain and inflammation through natural means, aligning with a holistic approach to health and wellness.

Herbal Poultices for Pain

Herbal poultices offer a time-honored method for addressing pain directly at its source, providing relief through the application of herbs in a form that allows their medicinal properties to be absorbed through the skin. Crafting an effective herbal poultice involves selecting the right herbs, preparing them properly, and applying them in a way that maximizes their therapeutic benefits. This section delves into the specifics of creating and using herbal poultices for pain relief, providing detailed guidance to ensure safety and efficacy.

To begin, select herbs known for their pain-relieving properties. Chamomile, for instance, is renowned for its anti-inflammatory and soothing effects, making it ideal for muscle pain or skin irritation. For joint pain or inflammation, turmeric, with its active compound curcumin, can be highly effective. Other herbs like ginger, known for its anti-inflammatory and circulatory benefits, can be used for a wide range of pain types, including arthritis and menstrual cramps.

Once you've selected the appropriate herb or combination of herbs, the next step is to prepare them for application. Fresh herbs should be finely chopped or ground to release their active compounds. If using dried herbs, they may need to be moistened with a small amount of hot water to rehydrate them, making them pliable and easy to apply. The goal is to create a paste-like consistency that can be spread over the affected area but is not so wet that it becomes runny.

For the base of the poultice, you can use a clean, thin cloth or gauze. Spread the herb paste evenly over the cloth, then fold it to encase the herbs completely. The poultice should then be applied directly to the skin over the area experiencing pain. To enhance the therapeutic effects, cover the poultice with plastic wrap to keep it moist and secure it with a bandage or medical tape. This also helps in maintaining contact with the skin and prevents staining of clothing or bedding.

The poultice can be left in place for up to 4 hours, depending on the severity of the pain and the specific herbs used. Some herbs, like turmeric, may cause staining of the skin or fabric, so it's important to consider this when determining the duration of application. For continuous relief, a fresh poultice can be applied as needed, allowing the skin to breathe between applications.

Warmth can sometimes enhance the effectiveness of a poultice, especially for conditions like muscle stiffness or cramps. Before applying the poultice, it can be gently warmed in a microwave for a few seconds or placed over a steaming pot of water, taking care not to overheat and risk burns. Always test the temperature before applying to the skin.

Materials Needed:
- Fresh or dried herbs (chamomile, turmeric, ginger)
- Mortar and pestle or a food processor for grinding herbs
- Hot water (if rehydrating dried herbs)
- Clean, thin cloth or gauze
- Plastic wrap
- Bandage or medical tape

Preparation and Application Steps:
1. Prepare the herbs by grinding or chopping to a fine consistency. Rehydrate dried herbs with a minimal amount of hot water to form a paste.
2. Spread the herb paste onto a clean cloth or gauze, then fold to encase the herbs.
3. Apply the poultice directly to the affected area, covering with plastic wrap and securing with a bandage or tape.
4. Leave in place for up to 4 hours, monitoring for any adverse reactions.
5. Remove and wash the area gently with warm water. Allow the skin to breathe before applying a new poultice if needed.

Safety Considerations:
- Conduct a patch test on a small area of skin before applying a poultice, especially if using herbs for the first time, to ensure no allergic reaction occurs.
- Consult with a healthcare provider before using herbal poultices, particularly for individuals who are pregnant, nursing, or have existing health conditions.
- Be mindful of the temperature of warmed poultices to prevent burns.

By incorporating herbal poultices into your approach to pain management, you can utilize the natural healing properties of herbs in a direct and effective manner. This method, rooted in ancient practices, offers a holistic alternative or complement to conventional pain relief methods, aligning with a commitment to natural wellness and self-care.

Chapter 4: Women's Health

Cramp Relief Teas for menstrual discomfort are a cornerstone of holistic family health, especially within the realm of women's wellness. The discomfort and pain associated with menstrual cramps can significantly disrupt daily activities and overall quality of life. However, the use of specific herbs in the preparation of teas can offer gentle, effective relief without the side effects often associated with over-the-counter medications.

Chamomile tea is renowned for its anti-inflammatory properties, which can help reduce the severity of menstrual cramps. The active compound in chamomile, bisabolol, works by relaxing the muscles of the uterus, thereby diminishing the intensity of cramp-induced pain. To prepare chamomile tea, steep 2-3 grams of dried chamomile flowers in 8 ounces of boiling water for 10-15 minutes. This allows for the full extraction of the herb's medicinal properties. For optimal results, it's recommended to begin drinking chamomile tea a week before the onset of menstruation and continue throughout the period as needed.

Ginger tea is another effective remedy for menstrual cramps, thanks to its potent anti-inflammatory and analgesic properties. Ginger works by inhibiting the synthesis of prostaglandins, compounds that play a key role in triggering the muscle contractions that cause menstrual pain. To make ginger tea, slice or grate 1-2 inches of fresh ginger root and simmer in 2 cups of water for 10-15 minutes. Strain the tea and add honey or lemon to taste if desired. Drinking ginger tea at the onset of cramps or even a few days before the menstrual cycle begins can significantly alleviate pain.

Peppermint tea, with its muscle-relaxing and pain-relieving effects, is another herbal tea that can be beneficial for those experiencing menstrual discomfort. The menthol in peppermint acts as a natural analgesic, providing relief from the throbbing pain associated with menstrual cramps. To prepare peppermint tea, steep 1 tablespoon of dried peppermint leaves in 8 ounces of boiling water for 7-10 minutes. Peppermint tea can be consumed as needed during menstruation to ease cramp pain and discomfort.

It's important to note that while these herbal teas are generally safe for most individuals, those with specific health conditions or who are pregnant should consult with a healthcare provider before incorporating them into their wellness routine. Additionally, the quality of herbs used can significantly impact the efficacy of the tea, so sourcing herbs from reputable suppliers is crucial.

In addition to the teas mentioned, there are other herbal remedies and supplements that can support women's health during menstruation, such as magnesium supplements and omega-3 fatty acids, which have been shown to reduce menstrual pain. However, the simplicity and accessibility of herbal teas make them an appealing first line of defense against menstrual cramps, aligning with the holistic approach to family wellness promoted throughout this guide.

Raspberry leaf tea is another invaluable addition to the natural apothecary for menstrual health. Often referred to as the "woman's herb," raspberry leaf contains fragarine and tannins, which are thought to strengthen and tone the uterine muscles, potentially easing menstrual cramps. To harness these benefits, steep 1-2 teaspoons of dried raspberry leaves in 8 ounces of boiling water for about 15 minutes. Starting this regimen a couple of days before the expected start of the menstrual cycle and continuing through the period may help reduce the severity of cramps.

Incorporating these herbal teas into a daily routine requires understanding the specific needs and responses of one's body. For instance, while some may find immediate relief with chamomile tea, others might benefit more from the cumulative effects of raspberry leaf tea over several cycles. It's also beneficial to alternate between different types of teas to prevent potential desensitization to their effects and to enjoy a variety of flavors.

For those new to using herbal remedies, it's advisable to start with lower concentrations of tea, gradually increasing the strength as needed and as one becomes familiar with how the body responds. This personalized approach ensures not only the effectiveness of the remedies but also minimizes the risk of adverse reactions.

Furthermore, lifestyle modifications such as regular exercise, stress management techniques like yoga or meditation, and a balanced diet rich in anti-inflammatory foods can complement the use of herbal teas for menstrual cramp relief. These holistic practices contribute to overall well-being and can enhance the body's natural ability to manage pain.

Lastly, maintaining a menstrual diary can be an insightful practice. Documenting the frequency, duration, intensity of cramps, and the remedies that provided relief can help identify patterns and tailor a more effective and personalized approach to managing menstrual discomfort.

The integration of these herbal teas and holistic practices into one's wellness routine embodies the essence of a family home apothecary. By fostering an environment of natural health and self-care, individuals can empower themselves and their families to lead healthier, more harmonious lives.

Herbal Support for Menstruation

Dong Quai, also known as Angelica Sinensis, has been a cornerstone in traditional Chinese medicine for thousands of years, specifically for its benefits in women's health and menstruation support. Dong Quai is often referred to as "female ginseng" for its ability to help regulate menstrual cycles and ease menstrual discomfort. It contains compounds that may act as phytoestrogens, helping to balance hormone levels in the body. For those looking to incorporate Dong Quai into their menstrual health regimen, it can be consumed in several forms, including capsules, tinctures, or tea. When preparing Dong Quai tea, it's recommended to use about 4-6 grams of the root per 8 ounces of water. Boil the root in water for 30 to 40 minutes, then strain and drink the tea. It is often advised to start taking Dong Quai a few days before the expected start of the menstrual period and continue through the first few days of the cycle.

Vitex, or Chaste Tree Berry (Vitex agnus-castus), is another herb with a long history of use in herbal medicine for regulating hormonal imbalances and supporting menstrual health. Vitex works by acting on the pituitary gland, which in turn can help to normalize the production of certain hormones, including progesterone. This normalization can alleviate symptoms associated with PMS and irregular menstrual cycles. Vitex is available in various forms, such as capsules, tinctures, and teas. For those opting for a tincture, the general recommendation is 20-40 drops in water, taken once daily in the morning. Consistency is key with Vitex, as it may take several months to notice significant changes in menstrual symptoms.

Evening Primrose Oil is rich in gamma-linolenic acid (GLA), an essential fatty acid that plays a crucial role in the regulation of hormonal balance. This oil has been widely studied for its effectiveness in reducing PMS symptoms, such as breast tenderness, feelings of depression, irritability, and swelling and bloating from fluid retention. To incorporate Evening Primrose Oil into a menstrual health routine, it is typically taken in capsule form, with a common dosage being 500-1000 mg daily. It's advisable to start with the lower end of the dosage range and adjust as needed based on symptom relief.

Magnesium supplements can also play a supportive role in menstrual health by reducing menstrual cramps and overall discomfort. Magnesium works by relaxing the smooth muscle of the uterus and reducing the prostaglandins that cause period pain. A dosage of 200-400 mg of magnesium daily is often recommended, starting two days before the onset of menstruation and continuing through the first few days of the cycle.

Materials Needed:

- Dong Quai root (for tea preparation)
- Vitex (Chaste Tree Berry) capsules or tincture
- Evening Primrose Oil capsules
- Magnesium supplements

Preparation and Application Steps:

1. For Dong Quai tea, measure 4-6 grams of the root. Boil in 8 ounces of water for 30-40 minutes, strain, and drink.
2. Vitex can be taken as a tincture or capsule. If using a tincture, add 20-40 drops to water and consume once daily in the morning.
3. Evening Primrose Oil capsules should be taken according to the dosage on the product label, typically 500-1000 mg daily.
4. Begin taking magnesium supplements two days before menstruation starts, continuing through the first few days, with a recommended dosage of 200-400 mg daily.

Safety Considerations:
- Always consult with a healthcare provider before introducing new supplements or herbs into your regimen, especially if you are pregnant, nursing, or have existing health conditions.
- Monitor for any adverse reactions when starting a new supplement, particularly if combining multiple herbal remedies.
- Consider the quality and source of the herbs and supplements, opting for products that have been third-party tested for purity and potency.

By integrating these herbal supports and supplements into a holistic approach to menstrual health, individuals can find natural relief from menstrual discomfort and achieve a greater sense of well-being throughout their menstrual cycle.

Cramp Relief Teas

Cinnamon Tea is another beneficial brew for those seeking relief from menstrual cramps. Cinnamon is known for its anti-inflammatory and antispasmodic properties, which can help soothe the uterine muscles and reduce the pain associated with menstrual cramps. To prepare cinnamon tea, add one cinnamon stick or one teaspoon of ground cinnamon to 8 ounces of boiling water. Allow it to steep for 10-15 minutes. For added flavor and benefits, a teaspoon of honey can be mixed into the tea. It's advisable to start drinking cinnamon tea a few days before the onset of menstruation to maximize its cramp-relieving effects.

Licorice Root Tea offers another herbal solution for menstrual discomfort. Licorice root has a long history of use in herbal medicine for its ability to mimic the effects of estrogen in the body, potentially easing menstrual symptoms. To make licorice root tea, steep 1-2 teaspoons of dried licorice root in 8 ounces of boiling water for 10-15 minutes. Due to its potent effects, licorice root tea should be consumed in moderation, with a recommended limit of one cup per day. Individuals with high blood pressure or those taking medication for heart disease should avoid licorice root or consult with a healthcare provider before consumption.

Fennel Tea is recognized for its antispasmodic and anti-inflammatory properties, making it an effective remedy for menstrual cramps. Fennel works by relaxing the muscles in the uterus, thereby reducing cramp intensity. To prepare fennel tea, crush 1-2 teaspoons of fennel seeds and steep in 8 ounces of boiling water for 10-15 minutes. Strain the seeds and drink the tea warm. For best results, begin consuming fennel tea a couple of days before the expected start of your period and continue as needed throughout menstruation.

Materials Needed:
- Cinnamon stick or ground cinnamon
- Dried licorice root
- Fennel seeds

- Honey (optional for flavor)
- Boiling water
- Teapot or cup for steeping
- Strainer (if using seeds or loose herbs)

Preparation and Application Steps:

1. For **Cinnamon Tea**, add one cinnamon stick or one teaspoon of ground cinnamon to a teapot or cup. Pour 8 ounces of boiling water over the cinnamon and allow to steep for 10-15 minutes. Strain if necessary and add honey to taste.
2. To make **Licorice Root Tea**, place 1-2 teaspoons of dried licorice root into a teapot or cup. Cover with 8 ounces of boiling water and steep for 10-15 minutes. Strain the licorice root before drinking. Limit consumption to one cup per day.
3. For **Fennel Tea**, crush 1-2 teaspoons of fennel seeds to release their oil. Place the crushed seeds in a teapot or cup and cover with 8 ounces of boiling water. Steep for 10-15 minutes, then strain the seeds. Drink the tea warm for best results.

Safety Considerations:

- Always consult with a healthcare provider before adding new herbal teas to your regimen, especially if you have existing health conditions or are taking medications.
- Pregnant women or those trying to conceive should exercise caution with herbal teas, particularly licorice root, due to its estrogen-mimicking effects.
- Monitor for any allergic reactions when trying a new herb for the first time.
- Ensure the quality of the herbs by sourcing them from reputable suppliers to avoid contamination with pesticides or heavy metals.

By integrating these cramp relief teas into your menstrual health routine, you can take a proactive step towards managing menstrual discomfort naturally. Each tea offers unique benefits, allowing you to customize your approach based on personal preference and the specific symptoms you experience. Remember, the key to effective relief is consistency and understanding how your body responds to different herbal remedies.

Balancing Hormones Naturally

Balancing hormones naturally involves leveraging the healing properties of specific herbs and supplements that have been recognized for their ability to support endocrine health. **Ashwagandha**, an adaptogenic herb, plays a pivotal role in regulating stress hormones, primarily cortisol, which can significantly impact menstrual health and overall hormonal balance. For optimal results, a standardized extract of Ashwagandha root, ranging from 300-500 mg, should be taken once or twice daily. It's important to select a product that specifies the concentration of withanolides, the active compounds, ensuring a potency of at least 5%.

Maca Root is another powerful adaptogen known for its ability to enhance stamina and energy, but it's also praised for its effects on hormonal balance. Maca works by nourishing the hypothalamus and pituitary glands, which are crucial for regulating the ovarian hormones estrogen and progesterone. Incorporating 1,500-3,000 mg of Maca root powder into your daily diet, either through capsules or by adding it to smoothies, can aid in achieving hormonal equilibrium. Ensure the Maca is gelatinized, a process that removes starch for improved digestibility and nutrient absorption.

Flaxseeds are rich in lignans and omega-3 fatty acids, both of which support hormonal balance by binding to excess estrogen in the body and promoting its elimination. Grinding 1-2 tablespoons of flaxseeds daily and adding them to meals not only ensures a dose of fiber but also aids in maintaining a healthy estrogen-progesterone ratio. It's critical to grind the flaxseeds freshly or store the ground seeds in a refrigerator to preserve their fatty acids from oxidation.

Omega-3 Supplements, such as fish oil or algae oil, provide essential fatty acids that are vital for hormone production and can reduce inflammation, which is often linked to hormonal imbalances. A daily intake of 500-1000 mg of EPA and DHA combined is recommended. When selecting an omega-3 supplement, look for products that have been third-party tested for purity and free from heavy metals and other contaminants.

Materials Needed:
- Ashwagandha root extract (300-500 mg capsules)
- Maca root powder or capsules (1,500-3,000 mg)
- Whole flaxseeds (to be ground)
- Omega-3 supplements (fish oil or algae oil, 500-1000 mg of EPA and DHA)

Preparation and Application Steps:
1. For **Ashwagandha**, take one 300-500 mg capsule once or twice daily, preferably with meals to enhance absorption. Verify the withanolide concentration to ensure potency.
2. **Maca Root** can be consumed in powder form by incorporating 1,500-3,000 mg into smoothies or foods daily. If using capsules, follow the dosage on the product label. Opt for gelatinized Maca for better digestion.
3. Grind 1-2 tablespoons of **flaxseeds** using a coffee grinder or spice mill. Add the freshly ground seeds to yogurt, oatmeal, or smoothies. Store any unused portion in the refrigerator.
4. Take an **Omega-3 supplement** daily, with a meal, to achieve a dosage of 500-1000 mg of EPA and DHA. Ensure the product's purity and absence of contaminants by selecting third-party tested supplements.

Safety Considerations:

- Consult with a healthcare provider before starting any new supplement, especially if you are taking medication, have a health condition, or are pregnant or breastfeeding.
- Monitor your body's response to new supplements, noting any adverse reactions or side effects.
- Quality and sourcing are paramount when selecting herbal supplements and omega-3s. Opt for reputable brands that provide transparent information about ingredient sourcing and third-party testing.
- Due to the estrogenic activity of flaxseeds, individuals with hormone-sensitive conditions should discuss their use with a healthcare provider.

Incorporating these natural supports into your daily regimen can assist in achieving a balanced hormonal state, contributing to improved menstrual health and overall well-being.

Natural Pregnancy and Postpartum Care

Red Raspberry Leaf Tea is highly regarded among herbal remedies for pregnancy care, known for its uterine strengthening properties. This tea is believed to aid in easier labor and recovery by toning the muscles of the uterus. For preparation, steep one tablespoon of dried red raspberry leaves in 8 ounces of boiling water for 10-15 minutes. It's advisable for pregnant women to start with one cup a day in the second trimester and gradually increase to three cups as they approach their due date.

Ginger Root is another invaluable herb for managing morning sickness, a common discomfort during the first trimester of pregnancy. Ginger works by soothing the digestive system and reducing nausea. To make ginger tea, slice about one inch of fresh ginger root and steep in boiling water for 10-15 minutes. Adding honey or lemon can enhance the flavor and provide additional benefits. Limit intake to 2-3 cups a day to avoid potential side effects.

Dates are nutritious fruits that have been studied for their role in promoting cervical dilation and reducing the need for induced labor. Eating 6 dates daily starting from the 36th week of pregnancy is recommended. Dates are high in natural sugars, fiber, potassium, and magnesium, all of which are beneficial for pregnancy health.

Dandelion Leaf Tea supports healthy fluid balance and kidney function during pregnancy. It is a gentle diuretic, helping to reduce edema or swelling commonly experienced in the later stages of pregnancy. To prepare, steep one teaspoon of dried dandelion leaves in 8 ounces of boiling water for 10 minutes. It's important to limit consumption to one cup per day and always consult with a healthcare provider before adding dandelion to your diet during pregnancy.

Postpartum Care focuses on recovery and replenishing the body after birth.

Nettle Tea is rich in iron, vitamins A, C, K, and calcium, making it an excellent beverage to support postpartum recovery and milk production in breastfeeding mothers. Prepare by steeping one tablespoon of dried nettle leaves in 8 ounces of boiling water for 10-15 minutes. Drinking one to two cups daily can help new mothers replenish vital nutrients.

Calendula Cream can be applied to perineal tears or C-section scars to promote healing due to its anti-inflammatory and antimicrobial properties. For application, gently rub a small amount of calendula cream on the affected area two to three times a day. Ensure the product is labeled safe for postpartum use and does not contain any harmful additives.

Omega-3 Supplements continue to be crucial in postpartum care, especially for supporting mood and reducing the risk of postpartum depression. A daily intake of 200-300 mg of DHA is recommended for breastfeeding mothers to support brain health in both mother and baby.

Materials Needed:
- Dried red raspberry leaves
- Fresh ginger root
- Dates
- Dried dandelion leaves
- Dried nettle leaves
- Calendula cream (labeled safe for postpartum use)
- Omega-3 supplements (with high DHA content)

Preparation and Application Steps:
1. For **Red Raspberry Leaf Tea**, steep one tablespoon of leaves in 8 ounces of boiling water for 10-15 minutes. Begin with one cup daily in the second trimester, increasing to three cups closer to the due date.
2. **Ginger Tea** preparation involves slicing one inch of ginger root, steeping in boiling water for 10-15 minutes, and optionally adding honey or lemon. Limit to 2-3 cups daily.
3. Consume **6 dates daily** starting from the 36th week of pregnancy.
4. Prepare **Dandelion Leaf Tea** by steeping one teaspoon of leaves in 8 ounces of boiling water for 10 minutes, with a recommended limit of one cup per day.
5. **Nettle Tea** can be made by steeping one tablespoon of dried nettle leaves in boiling water for 10-15 minutes, with a recommended intake of one to two cups daily for postpartum recovery.
6. Apply **Calendula Cream** gently on perineal tears or C-section scars two to three times daily, ensuring the product's safety for postpartum use.
7. **Omega-3 Supplements** should be taken daily, with a focus on 200-300 mg of DHA for breastfeeding mothers.

Safety Considerations:
- Consultation with a healthcare provider is essential before starting any new herbal remedy or supplement during pregnancy and postpartum, especially for those with existing health conditions or on medication.

- Monitoring for any allergic reactions or side effects when trying new herbs or supplements is crucial for the safety of both mother and baby.
- Quality and sourcing of herbs and supplements should be carefully considered, opting for products tested for purity and free from contaminants.

Safe Herbs for Pregnancy

Peppermint Leaf Tea is renowned for its ability to alleviate morning sickness and digestive discomfort, common issues during pregnancy. To prepare peppermint leaf tea, add one tablespoon of dried peppermint leaves to 8 ounces of boiling water. Steep for 5-10 minutes before straining. This herb's calming effect on the stomach makes it a gentle, effective remedy for nausea. Limit intake to 1-2 cups per day to avoid overconsumption, as excessive use can lead to heartburn in some individuals.

Lemon Balm Tea offers a soothing, mild sedative effect beneficial for stress and anxiety, which some expectant mothers may experience. Brew lemon balm tea by adding two teaspoons of dried lemon balm leaves to 8 ounces of boiling water. Allow it to steep for 10 minutes. Lemon balm can help improve sleep quality and reduce anxiety when consumed in moderation. It's recommended to drink one cup in the evening to aid relaxation.

Materials Needed:
- Dried peppermint leaves
- Dried lemon balm leaves
- Boiling water
- Teapot or cup for steeping
- Strainer

Preparation and Application Steps:
1. For **Peppermint Leaf Tea**, place one tablespoon of dried peppermint leaves into a teapot or cup. Pour 8 ounces of boiling water over the leaves and allow to steep for 5-10 minutes. Strain the leaves before drinking. Begin with one cup per day, adjusting to a maximum of two if necessary.
2. To make **Lemon Balm Tea**, add two teaspoons of dried lemon balm leaves to a teapot or cup. Cover with 8 ounces of boiling water and steep for 10 minutes. Strain the leaves and enjoy one cup in the evening for its calming effects.

Safety Considerations:
- While peppermint and lemon balm teas are generally considered safe during pregnancy, it's crucial to consult with a healthcare provider before incorporating them into your daily routine, especially if you have a history of miscarriages or other pregnancy-related concerns.

- Start with a lower quantity of herbs and gradually increase to the recommended amount to assess your body's tolerance.
- Be aware of the quality of herbs used; choose organic when possible to avoid exposure to pesticides and ensure the purity of the tea.
- Monitor for any adverse reactions, such as heartburn or allergic responses, and reduce consumption or discontinue use if any negative symptoms occur.

Chamomile Tea is another herb often recommended for its calming properties, which can help manage insomnia and stress during pregnancy. However, due to its potential to act as a uterine stimulant, it should be used with caution. If choosing to consume chamomile tea, limit it to one small cup occasionally, and not as a regular part of your daily routine. Always prioritize consulting with a healthcare provider before adding chamomile or any new herb to your regimen during pregnancy.

Materials Needed:
- Dried chamomile flowers
- Boiling water
- Teapot or cup for steeping
- Strainer

Preparation and Application Steps:
1. To prepare **Chamomile Tea**, add one teaspoon of dried chamomile flowers to a cup or teapot. Pour 8 ounces of boiling water over the flowers and steep for 5 minutes. Strain the flowers and consume the tea sparingly, not exceeding one small cup on occasion.

Safety Considerations:
- Given chamomile's potential effects on the uterus, it's imperative to seek advice from a healthcare professional before including it in your diet during pregnancy.
- Start with a minimal amount to test your body's reaction before proceeding with consumption.
- As with all herbs, ensure chamomile is sourced from a reputable supplier to guarantee quality and safety.

By carefully selecting and preparing these herbal teas, you can harness natural remedies to support your well-being throughout pregnancy. Remember, moderation is key, and consulting with a healthcare provider is essential to ensure the safety and health of both you and your baby.

Herbal Remedies for Postpartum Recovery

Continuing with the focus on herbal remedies for postpartum recovery, it is essential to address the common concern of lactation support for breastfeeding mothers. Fenugreek seeds are widely recognized for their galactagogue properties, which can enhance milk production. To prepare fenugreek tea, one should steep one teaspoon of crushed fenugreek seeds in 8 ounces of boiling water for 10-15 minutes. It is recommended to consume one cup of this tea two to three times a day. However, it is crucial to monitor for signs of gastrointestinal upset in both mother and baby, as fenugreek can cause such side effects in some individuals.

Another vital aspect of postpartum recovery is managing hormonal fluctuations that can lead to mood swings and postpartum depression. St. John's Wort is an herb known for its mood-stabilizing properties. For those considering this remedy, a standard dosage is to take 300 mg of St. John's Wort extract three times daily. This regimen should only be started under the guidance of a healthcare provider, especially for breastfeeding mothers, as the active compounds can be transferred to the baby through breast milk.

To support overall vitality and energy levels, which can be significantly depleted in the postpartum period, incorporating Shatavari root into the diet can be beneficial. Shatavari, an adaptogenic herb, supports the body's resilience to stress and aids in balancing hormones. A simple way to consume Shatavari is by taking 500 mg of the powdered root once or twice daily, mixed into a glass of warm milk or water. This practice can help rejuvenate the body and promote a sense of well-being.

Addressing physical recovery, particularly for mothers who have experienced a vaginal delivery, a sitz bath infused with witch hazel and lavender can provide soothing relief to perineal areas. To prepare the bath, fill a basin with warm water and add one cup of witch hazel and five to ten drops of lavender essential oil. Sitting in this mixture for 15 minutes can help reduce inflammation and promote healing of tears or episiotomies.

Lastly, for mothers experiencing hair loss, a common postpartum issue due to hormonal changes, a scalp massage with rosemary essential oil can stimulate hair growth and improve scalp health. Mix three to five drops of rosemary essential oil with a tablespoon of a carrier oil such as coconut or almond oil. Gently massage this blend into the scalp for several minutes before washing hair as usual. This treatment can be applied two to three times a week.

Materials Needed:
- Fenugreek seeds
- St. John's Wort extract
- Shatavari powder
- Witch hazel
- Lavender essential oil
- Rosemary essential oil
- Carrier oil (coconut or almond oil)
- Boiling water
- Basin for sitz bath

Preparation and Application Steps:

1. For **Fenugreek Tea**, crush one teaspoon of fenugreek seeds and steep in 8 ounces of boiling water for 10-15 minutes. Consume two to three times daily, observing for any adverse reactions.
2. **St. John's Wort** extract should be taken as 300 mg three times daily, under the supervision of a healthcare provider to ensure safety for both mother and baby.
3. **Shatavari Powder** can be taken by mixing 500 mg into warm milk or water once or twice daily to support hormonal balance and vitality.
4. Prepare a **Sitz Bath** by filling a basin with warm water, adding one cup of witch hazel and five to ten drops of lavender essential oil, and soaking for 15 minutes to aid in perineal recovery.
5. For **Scalp Massage**, blend three to five drops of rosemary essential oil with a tablespoon of carrier oil and massage into the scalp to promote hair growth and scalp health.

Safety Considerations:

- Always consult with a healthcare provider before beginning any new herbal supplement, especially during the postpartum period and while breastfeeding, to ensure the safety of both mother and baby.
- Be mindful of the quality of herbs and essential oils used, opting for organic and pure products to avoid exposure to pesticides and adulterants.
- Observe for any allergic reactions or side effects when trying new remedies, discontinuing use immediately if any adverse symptoms occur.
- Ensure that any bath or topical application is tested for temperature and sensitivity on a small skin area before full use to prevent burns or irritation.

Chapter 5: Children's Health

For addressing **common childhood ailments** such as **colds**, **coughs**, and **fevers**, natural remedies can be both effective and gentle. **Echinacea** is a powerful herb known for its immune-boosting properties. To prepare Echinacea tea for a child, steep half a teaspoon of dried Echinacea in 8 ounces of boiling water for 10-15 minutes. Strain and cool the tea to a suitable temperature before giving it to the child. A dosage of up to 2-3 cups per day for children over two years old is generally considered safe for short-term use during the onset of cold symptoms.

Honey and Lemon Syrup serves as a soothing remedy for coughs and sore throats. Mix one tablespoon of raw, organic honey with two teaspoons of fresh lemon juice. This mixture can be given to children over one year old, up to three times a day. Honey is not recommended for children under one year due to the risk of botulism.

For **fevers**, **Linden Flower Tea** is a gentle option that promotes sweating and helps lower body temperature naturally. Use one teaspoon of dried linden flowers per 8 ounces of boiling water, steeping for 15 minutes. Ensure the tea is cooled to a safe drinking temperature before offering it to your child. It's suitable for children over the age of two, and can be given 2-3 times daily during feverish conditions.

To support **digestive health** and alleviate **stomach upsets**, **Ginger Tea** can be beneficial. Slice a quarter-inch piece of fresh ginger and steep in 8 ounces of boiling water for 10-15 minutes. For children, offering a quarter to half a cup of this tea can help soothe nausea or digestive discomfort. Always allow the tea to cool to a safe temperature before serving.

Chamomile Tea is well-known for its calming effects and can be particularly useful for children experiencing **sleep difficulties** or **anxiety**. Prepare the tea by steeping one teaspoon of dried chamomile flowers in 8 ounces of boiling water for about 5-10 minutes. For young children, a half-cup of tea before bedtime can promote relaxation and sleep.

Materials Needed:

- Dried Echinacea
- Raw, organic honey
- Fresh lemon
- Dried linden flowers
- Fresh ginger root
- Dried chamomile flowers
- Boiling water

Preparation Steps:

1. For **Echinacea Tea**, steep half a teaspoon of dried Echinacea in 8 ounces of boiling water for 10-15 minutes. Strain and cool before serving.
2. To make **Honey and Lemon Syrup**, mix one tablespoon of honey with two teaspoons of fresh lemon juice. Administer up to three times a day to children over one year old.
3. Prepare **Linden Flower Tea** by steeping one teaspoon of dried linden flowers in 8 ounces of boiling water for 15 minutes. Cool to a safe temperature before offering to your child.
4. For **Ginger Tea**, steep a quarter-inch slice of fresh ginger in 8 ounces of boiling water for 10-15 minutes. Serve a quarter to half a cup to help with digestive issues.
5. **Chamomile Tea** can be made by steeping one teaspoon of dried chamomile flowers in 8 ounces of boiling water for 5-10 minutes. Offer a half-cup before bedtime to aid sleep.

Safety Considerations:
- Always consult with a healthcare provider before introducing new herbs or supplements to your child's regimen, especially if your child is under the age of two or has existing health conditions.
- Begin with small doses to monitor for any allergic reactions or adverse effects.
- Ensure all teas are cooled to a safe temperature to prevent burns.
- Honey should not be given to children under one year of age to avoid the risk of botulism.
- Quality and purity of herbs are crucial; opt for organic products when possible to minimize exposure to pesticides and contaminants.

Gentle Remedies for Childhood Ailments

For **skin irritations** and **rashes** commonly experienced by children, **Aloe Vera Gel** is a soothing and healing remedy. Directly apply the gel from an aloe vera leaf to the affected area. The gel should be harvested by slicing a leaf open and scooping out the clear, inner gel. Apply a thin layer of this gel to the child's skin irritation, ensuring the area is clean and dry beforehand. Aloe vera is known for its cooling properties and can be applied 2-3 times daily until the irritation improves.

Calendula Cream is another effective treatment for skin issues, including diaper rash and eczema. To use, apply a small amount of calendula cream to the affected area after each diaper change or bath, ensuring the skin is dry. Calendula has natural anti-inflammatory and healing properties, making it ideal for sensitive skin.

For **minor burns** and **scrapes**, **Honey** can be used as a natural antiseptic. Apply a thin layer of raw, organic honey to a clean, minor wound or burn to help prevent infection and promote healing. Cover lightly with a sterile bandage. Honey's antibacterial properties make it suitable for minor, superficial skin injuries.

Lavender Essential Oil diluted in a carrier oil such as coconut oil can be gently applied to areas of **insect bites** to reduce inflammation and soothe itchiness. Mix one drop of lavender essential oil with one teaspoon of carrier oil and apply a small amount to the bite. Lavender's anti-inflammatory and analgesic properties can provide immediate relief from insect bites and stings.

Materials Needed:
- Aloe vera leaf
- Calendula cream
- Raw, organic honey
- Lavender essential oil
- Carrier oil (coconut or almond oil)

Preparation and Application Steps:
1. For **Aloe Vera Gel**, slice an aloe vera leaf lengthwise and scoop out the gel. Apply directly to the skin irritation or rash 2-3 times daily.
2. **Calendula Cream** should be applied in a thin layer to clean, dry skin affected by rash or irritation, after each diaper change or bath for babies and toddlers.
3. To use **Honey** for minor burns or scrapes, apply a thin layer to the clean wound and cover with a sterile bandage. Change daily.
4. For **Lavender Essential Oil**, dilute one drop in one teaspoon of carrier oil and apply a small amount to the insect bite to reduce itchiness and inflammation.

Safety Considerations:
- Always perform a patch test on a small area of the child's skin before applying a new product or remedy to ensure there is no allergic reaction.
- Do not apply honey to wounds in children under one year of age due to the risk of botulism.
- Consult with a healthcare provider before using any new treatment on your child, especially if they have pre-existing health conditions or allergies.
- Ensure the purity and quality of all ingredients used, opting for organic and natural products whenever possible to minimize exposure to harmful chemicals and additives.
- Monitor the child's reaction to the treatment closely, discontinuing use and seeking medical advice if any adverse reactions occur.

Herbal Solutions for Colic

Colic in infants can be a distressing condition, characterized by periods of intense, unexplained crying. Natural herbal remedies can offer gentle relief for this common ailment. When considering herbal solutions, it's crucial to use safe, mild herbs that are appropriate for infants. One such remedy is **Fennel Seed Tea**, known for its antispasmodic and gas-relieving properties.

Materials Needed:

- Organic fennel seeds
- Purified water
- Strainer or cheesecloth
- Bottle or dropper for feeding

Preparation Steps:

1. Crush **one teaspoon of organic fennel seeds** using a mortar and pestle to release their volatile oils. The crushing process should be gentle, aiming to slightly crack the seeds rather than turning them into a powder.
2. Boil **8 ounces of purified water** and then add the crushed fennel seeds. Cover and simmer on low heat for 10 minutes. This slow simmering process allows for the extraction of the seeds' beneficial compounds without destroying them.
3. Remove from heat and let the tea cool to room temperature. Strain the tea using a fine strainer or cheesecloth to remove all seed particles. It's essential to ensure that the tea is completely free of any small seeds or fragments to prevent any choking hazard.
4. Store the strained tea in a clean bottle or dropper. The tea can be stored in the refrigerator for up to 48 hours. Before use, warm the tea gently by placing the bottle in a bowl of warm water. Do not microwave, as this can create hot spots that might burn the baby's mouth.

Application Steps:

- For infants, administer **1 teaspoon (5 ml) of fennel tea**, up to three times a day. Use a clean dropper or add it to the baby's bottle. The dosage should not exceed 3 teaspoons in a 24-hour period.
- Observe the infant for any signs of allergic reaction or discomfort after administration, such as hives, rash, or increased distress. Although rare, it's important to monitor and discontinue use if any adverse reactions occur.

Safety Considerations:

- Always consult with a pediatrician before introducing any new remedy to an infant's diet, especially for babies under six months old.
- Ensure that all equipment used in the preparation of the tea is sterilized to prevent any risk of infection.
- Quality of herbs is paramount. Opt for organic fennel seeds to minimize the infant's exposure to pesticides and other chemicals.
- Start with the smallest dose possible to assess the baby's tolerance to the herbal remedy.

Fennel Seed Tea is a time-honored remedy for colic, offering a natural option to soothe and comfort infants experiencing colic symptoms. Its effectiveness lies in its ability to relax the smooth muscles of the gastrointestinal tract, thereby reducing gas and spasms that can lead to intense crying episodes. By adhering to the preparation and safety guidelines outlined, parents can provide a gentle, herbal solution to help alleviate their baby's colic symptoms, ensuring a more peaceful environment for both the infant and the family.

Natural Remedies for Skin Irritations

Oatmeal Baths are another time-tested remedy, particularly effective for soothing itchy, irritated skin caused by chickenpox, eczema, or sunburns. To prepare an oatmeal bath for a child, grind 1 cup of plain, unflavored oats in a food processor or blender until they reach a fine, powdery consistency. This powder should then be dispersed in a bathtub filled with lukewarm water, ensuring the water is not too hot to prevent further irritation of the skin. Stir the water to ensure the oatmeal is evenly distributed. Have the child soak in the oatmeal bath for 15-20 minutes. Avoid using any soap during the bath, as it can strip the skin of its natural oils and exacerbate dryness. After the bath, gently pat the child's skin dry with a soft towel, avoiding rubbing, which can irritate the skin further. Applying a moisturizer that is free from fragrances and dyes immediately after patting the skin dry can help lock in moisture and protect the skin barrier.

For dealing with diaper rash, Coconut Oil serves as an excellent natural remedy due to its antifungal and antibacterial properties. After each diaper change, clean the baby's bottom with warm water and pat dry. Apply a thin layer of virgin coconut oil to the affected area. Virgin coconut oil is preferred due to its minimal processing, ensuring that its beneficial properties are intact. This oil not only helps to soothe the skin but also creates a barrier that protects against moisture, reducing the risk of further irritation.

Tea Tree Oil, diluted in a carrier oil, can be effective for older children suffering from skin irritations such as acne. It is important to note that tea tree oil must be diluted before application to the skin to prevent irritation. A recommended dilution is 1-2 drops of tea tree oil in 1 tablespoon of carrier oil, such as jojoba or sweet almond oil. Apply the mixture directly to the affected area with a cotton swab once daily. Due to its potent antimicrobial properties, tea tree oil can help reduce inflammation and clear up blemishes. However, it's crucial to conduct a patch test on a small area of the skin before full application to ensure there is no allergic reaction.

Witch Hazel, applied with a cotton ball to areas of inflammation or insect bites, can provide immediate relief due to its astringent and anti-inflammatory properties. This natural remedy is particularly useful for soothing mosquito bites and reducing the urge to scratch, which can further damage the skin. Witch Hazel should be used in its pure form, without alcohol, to avoid drying out the skin.

When utilizing these natural remedies, it's essential to observe the child's skin reaction closely. While these treatments are generally safe, every child's skin is unique, and what works for one may not work for another. Discontinue use immediately if any remedy causes redness, irritation, or an allergic reaction and consult a healthcare provider. The goal is to provide gentle, effective relief that supports the skin's natural healing process without the use of harsh chemicals or medications that can lead to other side effects. By choosing natural remedies, parents can feel confident in their approach to managing common skin irritations in children, fostering a healthy, happy environment for their family's wellness journey.

Boosting Children's Immunity Naturally

Incorporating **Vitamin D** into a child's routine is pivotal for enhancing their immune system. The body synthesizes Vitamin D primarily through direct sunlight exposure, which can be challenging during winter months or in regions with limited sunlight. For children, a daily exposure of 10-15 minutes to sunlight, preferably in the early morning to avoid the harsh rays, can significantly contribute to their Vitamin D levels. However, during less sunny seasons, consider supplementing with Vitamin D drops or foods fortified with Vitamin D, such as certain cereals, orange juice, and dairy products. The recommended dietary allowance (RDA) for Vitamin D varies by age, but generally, children aged 1-13 years should aim for 600 International Units (IU) per day.

Probiotics play a crucial role in maintaining gut health, which is directly linked to the immune system's effectiveness. Foods rich in probiotics, like yogurt, kefir, and fermented foods (sauerkraut, kimchi), should be incorporated into a child's diet. For children averse to these flavors, probiotic supplements designed for pediatric use can be an alternative. When selecting a probiotic supplement, look for one that contains a variety of strains and has a CFU (colony-forming units) count appropriate for children.

Zinc is an essential mineral that supports the immune system's ability to fight off illness. Foods high in zinc include beans, nuts, whole grains, and dairy products. The RDA for zinc in children ranges from 3 mg/day for infants to 8 mg/day for children aged 4-8 years. In cases where dietary intake may not meet these needs, a zinc supplement can be considered, but it's important to consult with a healthcare provider to determine the appropriate dosage.

Elderberry syrup is renowned for its immune-boosting properties and has been used for centuries to prevent and fight off colds and flu. Elderberry is rich in antioxidants and vitamins that can help reduce inflammation, lessen stress, and protect the heart. For children, elderberry syrup can be given at the first sign of immune distress. Ensure that the elderberry product chosen is specifically formulated for children, free from harmful additives, and does not exceed the recommended dosage on the product label.

Hydration is fundamental for overall health and aids in the proper functioning of the immune system. Encourage children to drink water throughout the day by providing them with a personal water bottle and setting reminders or making it a fun challenge to finish their water by the end of the day. Avoid sugary drinks as they can suppress the immune system and lead to other health issues.

Sleep is when the body repairs itself and strengthens its immune response. Establishing a consistent bedtime routine that ensures children get the recommended amount of sleep for their age is crucial. For toddlers aged 1-2 years, 11-14 hours of sleep (including naps) are recommended, while children aged 3-5 years should get 10-13 hours, and those aged 6-13 years need 9-11 hours of sleep per night.

Physical Activity should be encouraged as it helps to boost the immune system by increasing blood circulation and reducing stress. Aim for at least 60 minutes of moderate to vigorous physical activity daily for children. Activities can include biking, hiking, playing sports, or simply playing outside.

Materials Needed:
- Vitamin D supplements (if necessary)
- Probiotic-rich foods or supplements
- Foods high in zinc or zinc supplements (consult healthcare provider)
- Elderberry syrup formulated for children
- Personal water bottles
- Tools to encourage physical activity (sports equipment, bicycles)

Preparation and Application Steps:
1. Ensure daily outdoor activity for natural sunlight exposure; morning hours are preferable.
2. Incorporate probiotic-rich foods into meals or select a child-friendly probiotic supplement.
3. Include zinc-rich foods in the diet; consult a healthcare provider if considering a zinc supplement.
4. Administer elderberry syrup according to product guidelines at the first sign of immune distress.
5. Promote hydration by making water readily available and limiting sugary drinks.
6. Establish a consistent bedtime routine to ensure adequate sleep.
7. Encourage daily physical activity suitable for the child's age and interests.

Safety Considerations:
- Always consult with a pediatric healthcare provider before introducing any supplements to a child's routine.
- Monitor for any allergic reactions when introducing new foods or supplements.
- Ensure any elderberry product is safe for pediatric use and does not contain honey if under one year of age.
- Practice sun safety by applying sunscreen during prolonged sun exposure.
- Ensure physical activities are age-appropriate and conducted in a safe environment.

Kid-Friendly Herbal Supplements

Incorporating **kid-friendly herbal supplements** into your child's wellness routine can be an effective way to support their immune system and overall health. When selecting herbal supplements, it's critical to choose products that are specifically designed for children, with appropriate dosages and formulations. Here are some guidelines and specific herbal supplements that can be beneficial for children:

"Selecting Herbal Supplements"

- **Quality and Purity**: Look for supplements that are certified organic, non-GMO, and free from artificial colors, flavors, and preservatives. Certifications from reputable organizations can provide assurance about the quality of the product.
- **Age-Appropriate Formulations**: Ensure the supplement is intended for children, with dosages adjusted for their age and weight. This information is usually provided on the product label.
- **Third-Party Testing**: Opt for products that have undergone third-party testing for potency and purity. This adds an extra layer of safety and ensures that the supplement contains what it claims to.

"Recommended Herbal Supplements"
- **Multivitamin and Mineral Supplements**: A broad-spectrum multivitamin designed for children can fill nutritional gaps in their diet. Look for a formula that includes essential vitamins and minerals, such as Vitamin C, Vitamin D, Zinc, and Iron, in child-appropriate dosages.
- **Echinacea**: Known for its immune-boosting properties, Echinacea can be particularly beneficial during cold and flu season. Liquid extracts or chewable tablets formulated for children can make administration easier. The typical dosage for children is a lower concentration, often specified on the product label.
- **Omega-3 Fatty Acids**: Essential for brain development and immune function, Omega-3 supplements derived from fish oil or algae are available in flavors and forms appealing to children, such as chewable soft gels or liquid.
- **Probiotics**: Supporting gut health with probiotics can enhance immune function. Choose a probiotic supplement with strains specifically researched for children's health. The CFU count should be suitable for children, and the product should include instructions for pediatric dosing.
- **Vitamin D**: Especially important in areas with limited sunlight exposure, Vitamin D supplements can support immune health, bone growth, and overall well-being. Drops are often the easiest form to administer to children, with dosages provided based on age and need.

"Administration Tips"
- **Incorporate into Routine**: Establish a consistent time for taking supplements, such as with breakfast, to create a routine.
- **Mix with Food or Drinks**: If the child is resistant to taking supplements, mixing liquid forms into a small amount of juice or food can help with administration.
- **Educate on Importance**: Explain to children in simple terms why they are taking the supplement and its benefits to their health.

"Safety Considerations"
- **Consult a Pediatrician**: Before starting any new supplement, it's important to discuss it with your child's healthcare provider, especially if your child has any health conditions or takes other medications.
- **Start with Low Doses**: Begin with the lowest recommended dose for your child's age group to assess tolerance.

- **Monitor for Reactions**: Keep an eye on any changes in your child's health or behavior that could indicate an adverse reaction to the supplement.

"Materials Needed"
- **Child-friendly Herbal Supplement**: Choose based on the specific need, such as immune support or nutritional supplementation.
- **Measuring Tool**: Use the measuring tool provided with liquid supplements for accurate dosing.
- **Journal**: Keeping a log of the supplements taken and any observed effects can be helpful for tracking tolerance and effectiveness.

By carefully selecting and administering herbal supplements designed for children, parents can support their child's health and immune system in a natural, holistic manner. Always prioritize safety by choosing high-quality, tested products and consulting healthcare professionals to ensure these supplements complement your child's health regimen effectively.

By scanning the QR code below

you can download your

Home Apothecary Video

and 3000 other Remedies

Chapter 6: Men's Health

In addressing **men's health**, focusing on **prostate health** and **enhancing vitality and energy** is crucial. A holistic approach incorporates specific herbs known for their beneficial effects on these areas.

"Prostate Health"
For **prostate health**, **Saw Palmetto** is a well-regarded herb. It's believed to help in reducing the symptoms of an enlarged prostate, a common condition known as benign prostatic hyperplasia (BPH). The active compounds in Saw Palmetto may help to inhibit the conversion of testosterone into dihydrotestosterone, a hormone associated with prostate enlargement.

Materials Needed:
- Saw Palmetto berries or extract
- Capsule machine if making your own capsules
- Dark, glass bottles if using liquid extract

Preparation and Application Steps:
1. **Saw Palmetto Extract**: For convenience, purchasing a high-quality, standardized Saw Palmetto extract is recommended. Look for products that specify the percentage of fatty acids, as these are the active components. The typical dosage is 160 mg twice daily of an extract containing 85-95% fatty acids.
2. **Homemade Saw Palmetto Capsules**: If you prefer to prepare your own, purchase dried Saw Palmetto berries. Grind them into a fine powder using a coffee grinder. Using a capsule machine, fill empty capsules with the powdered berries. Follow the manufacturer's instructions for dosage, generally aligning with the extract dosage guidelines.

"Enhancing Vitality and Energy"
To **enhance vitality and energy**, incorporating **Ashwagandha** and **Ginseng** can be particularly effective. Both herbs are adaptogens, which means they help the body resist stressors of all kinds, whether physical, chemical, or biological.

Materials Needed:
- Ashwagandha root powder
- Ginseng root (American or Panax variety)
- Mortar and pestle or a grinder
- Capsule machine for homemade capsules
- Teapot and strainer for teas

Preparation and Application Steps:

1. **Ashwagandha**: This can be taken as a powder, in capsule form, or as a tea. For the powder, a common dose is about 1/4 to 1/2 teaspoon once or twice a day, mixed into a smoothie or milk. For making capsules, follow the process similar to Saw Palmetto, adjusting the dosage according to the package or a healthcare provider's recommendation.
2. **Ginseng Tea**: Slice 1 to 2 grams of Ginseng root thinly. Boil in 8 ounces of water for 15 minutes. Strain and drink once daily. Ginseng can also be taken as a capsule or extract, with dosages varying based on the product's concentration.

Safety Considerations:
- Always consult with a healthcare provider before starting any new supplement, especially for those with existing health conditions or those taking medications, as interactions can occur.
- Begin with the lower dosage range for any supplement and observe your body's response before increasing.
- For Saw Palmetto, while generally considered safe, some might experience mild side effects like stomach discomfort. It's important to monitor for any adverse reactions.
- Ashwagandha and Ginseng should be used cautiously by those with thyroid conditions, as they can influence hormone levels.
- Ensure the purity and quality of all herbs and supplements by purchasing from reputable sources.

By integrating these herbs into a daily routine, men can support their prostate health and enhance overall vitality and energy. This approach aligns with the book's emphasis on natural, holistic remedies for family wellness, offering practical and scientifically supported methods to improve men's health.

Natural Support for Prostate Health

Continuing with the holistic approach to **men's health**, particularly focusing on **prostate health**, it's essential to integrate certain dietary and lifestyle changes alongside the use of **herbal remedies**. The goal is to support and maintain prostate health naturally, reducing the risk of common conditions such as benign prostatic hyperplasia (BPH) and prostatitis. Here are specific strategies, foods, and herbs that have been recognized for their potential benefits in supporting prostate health.

Dietary Adjustments for Prostate Health:
- **Increase the intake of fruits and vegetables**: Aim for a colorful variety, focusing on those rich in antioxidants such as tomatoes, which contain lycopene, a compound thought to support prostate health. Cruciferous vegetables like broccoli, Brussels sprouts, and cabbage are also beneficial due to their sulforaphane content.
- **Select healthy fats**: Incorporate sources of omega-3 fatty acids found in fish like salmon, mackerel, and sardines. These fats are known for their anti-inflammatory properties.

- **Choose plant-based proteins**: Legumes, such as beans and lentils, are excellent sources of protein and fiber, which can help in maintaining a healthy weight, a factor in reducing prostate health risks.
- **Stay hydrated**: Drinking plenty of water is crucial for overall health and can help in maintaining proper urinary function.

Herbs and Supplements for Prostate Health:
- **Saw Palmetto**: As previously mentioned, Saw Palmetto is widely used for BPH symptoms. It's thought to work by inhibiting the enzyme 5-alpha-reductase, reducing the conversion of testosterone to dihydrotestosterone (DHT), a hormone linked to prostate enlargement.
- **Pygeum**: Derived from the bark of the African cherry tree, Pygeum has been used in traditional medicine for urinary issues. It's believed to contain compounds that can help reduce inflammation and improve urinary symptoms associated with an enlarged prostate.
- **Stinging Nettle**: Often used in combination with Saw Palmetto, Stinging Nettle may help alleviate symptoms of BPH. It's thought to work by inhibiting the binding of sex hormone-binding globulin to prostate cells, which may reduce the proliferation of prostate cells.
- **Pumpkin Seeds**: Rich in zinc, a mineral important for prostate health, pumpkin seeds can be a beneficial addition to the diet. They may help in reducing BPH symptoms and improving urinary function.

Lifestyle Modifications:
- **Regular Exercise**: Maintaining regular physical activity can help in managing weight and reducing the risk of prostate issues. Aim for at least 150 minutes of moderate-intensity exercise per week.
- **Stress Management**: Chronic stress can negatively impact health, including prostate health. Practices such as meditation, yoga, and deep-breathing exercises can be effective in managing stress.
- **Adequate Sleep**: Ensuring sufficient sleep is vital for overall health and can support the body's natural healing processes, including those related to the prostate.

Preparation and Application Steps for Herbal Remedies:
1. **Saw Palmetto Extract**: Opt for a standardized extract and follow the recommended dosage on the product label, typically 160 mg twice daily.
2. **Pygeum**: Available as capsules or tinctures, follow the dosage guidelines provided by the manufacturer.
3. **Stinging Nettle**: Can be consumed as a tea, capsule, or tincture. If opting for tea, steep 1-2 teaspoons of dried nettle leaves in boiling water for 10 minutes. Drink up to 3 cups daily.
4. **Pumpkin Seeds**: Can be eaten raw, roasted, or added to salads and smoothies. Aim for a handful daily to reap the benefits.

Safety Considerations:
- Always consult with a healthcare provider before starting any new supplement, particularly for those with existing health conditions or taking medications.
- Monitor for any side effects or interactions with other medications and report them to your healthcare provider.

- Be cautious with dosages, especially when combining multiple supplements, to avoid potential adverse effects.

By adopting these dietary, lifestyle, and herbal strategies, men can take proactive steps toward maintaining prostate health. It's important to approach this holistically, integrating these practices into a comprehensive lifestyle plan for optimal wellness.

Enhancing Vitality and Energy

In the pursuit of **enhancing vitality and energy** in men's health, integrating **Maca Root** and **Rhodiola Rosea** alongside lifestyle modifications can significantly contribute to improved wellness. These herbs have been recognized for their capacity to support stamina, reduce fatigue, and enhance mental clarity, making them invaluable components of a holistic approach to men's vitality.

Maca Root, traditionally used for its energizing and stamina-increasing properties, is available in powder form, capsules, or as a liquid extract. A common starting dosage is 1,500 to 3,000 mg per day for capsules, or for the powder, 1 tablespoon mixed into smoothies or beverages. It's essential to start with a lower dosage, assessing tolerance before gradually increasing.

Rhodiola Rosea, known for its adaptogenic properties, helps the body adapt to and resist physical, chemical, and environmental stress. For Rhodiola, the recommended dosage often starts at 100 to 300 mg per day when using an extract standardized to 1% salidroside or 3% rosavins. It's best taken in the morning, with or without food, to avoid potential interference with sleep.

Materials Needed:
- Maca root powder or capsules
- Rhodiola Rosea extract, standardized to salidroside or rosavins
- Measuring spoon for powder dosages
- Water or beverage for mixing Maca powder

Preparation and Application Steps:
1. **Maca Powder**: If using powder, incorporate 1 tablespoon of Maca into a morning smoothie or beverage. Evaluate how your body responds to this initial amount, and consider increasing the dosage gradually, not exceeding 3 tablespoons per day.
2. **Maca Capsules**: For those preferring capsules, follow the manufacturer's recommended dosage, starting with the lower end of the dosage range.
3. **Rhodiola Rosea**: Begin with 100 mg of Rhodiola extract in the morning. Observe your body's response for a week, and if well-tolerated, the dosage can be increased, not exceeding 300 mg per day. Due to its energizing effects, Rhodiola is best taken earlier in the day.

Safety Considerations:

- Consultation with a healthcare provider is crucial before starting any new supplement regimen, especially for individuals with existing health conditions or those on medication.
- Monitor for any adverse reactions when introducing these supplements, and adjust dosages as necessary.
- Pregnant or nursing women should avoid these supplements due to insufficient research on their safety in these populations.
- Individuals with hormone-sensitive conditions should be cautious with Maca, as it may act as an endocrine modulator.

Lifestyle Modifications for Enhanced Vitality:

- **Regular Physical Activity**: Engage in at least 30 minutes of moderate exercise most days of the week to boost energy levels and overall health.
- **Balanced Diet**: Focus on nutrient-rich foods, including whole grains, lean proteins, healthy fats, and a variety of fruits and vegetables to support energy levels.
- **Adequate Hydration**: Drink plenty of water throughout the day to prevent dehydration, which can lead to fatigue.
- **Quality Sleep**: Aim for 7-9 hours of quality sleep per night to support recovery and energy levels.
- **Stress Management**: Incorporate stress-reduction techniques such as meditation, deep breathing exercises, or yoga into your daily routine to help manage stress levels, which can impact energy and vitality.

By incorporating Maca and Rhodiola Rosea into a lifestyle that prioritizes balanced nutrition, regular physical activity, adequate hydration, quality sleep, and effective stress management, men can enhance their vitality and energy levels. This holistic approach aligns with the book's emphasis on natural remedies and lifestyle modifications to support family wellness, offering practical and scientifically supported methods to improve men's health.

Chapter 7: Aging Gracefully

For those seeking to age gracefully, the inclusion of **Ginkgo Biloba** and **Turmeric** in one's daily regimen can offer significant benefits. These herbs are renowned for their ability to enhance cognitive function and reduce inflammation, respectively, which are common concerns as we age.

Ginkgo Biloba has been extensively studied for its potential to improve blood circulation and support brain health. This herb works by dilating blood vessels and reducing the stickiness of blood platelets, thus improving blood flow to the brain. Improved circulation can lead to better cognitive function and has been linked to a reduction in symptoms associated with cognitive decline.

Materials Needed:
- Ginkgo Biloba leaves or standardized extract
- Capsule machine for homemade capsules or a teapot for brewing tea

Preparation and Application Steps:
1. **Ginkgo Biloba Tea**: To prepare tea, steep 1-2 teaspoons of dried Ginkgo leaves in hot water for about 10 minutes. Strain and enjoy the tea once or twice daily.
2. **Ginkgo Biloba Capsules**: For those preferring capsules, using a standardized extract containing 24% flavone glycosides is recommended. The typical dosage is 120-240 mg per day, divided into two or three doses.

Turmeric, known for its active compound curcumin, offers powerful anti-inflammatory and antioxidant properties. Curcumin can help in reducing inflammation throughout the body, including the brain, and is thought to slow down age-related cognitive decline. Turmeric can be incorporated into the diet in various ways, from adding it to foods to taking it as a supplement.

Materials Needed:
- Turmeric powder or curcumin supplements
- Black pepper (to enhance absorption)
- Oil (for cooking with turmeric)

Preparation and Application Steps:
1. **Turmeric in Cooking**: Incorporate turmeric powder into your daily cooking, adding it to soups, stews, rice, or vegetable dishes. Combine with a pinch of black pepper to enhance the absorption of curcumin.
2. **Turmeric Golden Milk**: Mix 1 teaspoon of turmeric powder with a cup of warm milk (dairy or plant-based), a pinch of black pepper, and a teaspoon of honey or maple syrup for sweetness. Drink this mixture once daily.

3. **Curcumin Supplements**: If opting for a supplement, look for products that contain piperine (black pepper extract) and follow the manufacturer's recommended dosage, usually around 500-2,000 mg of curcumin per day.

Safety Considerations:
- Ginkgo Biloba may interact with blood thinners and other medications. Consult with a healthcare provider before starting, especially if you are on medication.
- Turmeric is generally safe but in high doses or supplement form, it can cause digestive upset or interact with medications. Always start with lower doses and consult a healthcare provider.
- Pregnant or nursing women should consult with a healthcare provider before taking these supplements.

In addition to these herbal remedies, maintaining a lifestyle that includes regular physical activity, a balanced diet rich in antioxidants, and adequate hydration is crucial for aging gracefully. Engaging in mental exercises and social activities can also support cognitive health and overall well-being. By integrating these practices and herbal remedies into your daily routine, you can support your body's natural aging process and maintain vitality and wellness into your later years.

Herbal Antioxidants for Longevity

To harness the power of herbal antioxidants for longevity, focusing on **Astaxanthin**, **Green Tea**, and **Resveratrol** provides a robust foundation. These compounds are celebrated for their potent antioxidant properties, which combat oxidative stress and may contribute to a longer, healthier life.

Astaxanthin is a keto-carotenoid found in certain algae, yeast, and seafood. It's one of the most powerful antioxidants available, significantly more potent than other carotenoids and vitamin E. Astaxanthin supports skin health, eye health, and cardiovascular health. For supplementation, look for **natural astaxanthin derived from Haematococcus pluvialis algae**. The recommended dosage is **4-12 mg per day**. When selecting a supplement, ensure it's from a reputable source to guarantee purity and effectiveness.

Green Tea, rich in catechins, particularly **epigallocatechin gallate (EGCG)**, offers extensive antioxidant benefits. These compounds help protect against cellular damage and have been linked to a reduction in the risk of certain chronic diseases. To incorporate green tea into your regimen, opt for **organic loose-leaf green tea** for the highest concentration of antioxidants. Aim to drink **2-3 cups daily**. If you prefer a supplement, seek out green tea extract standardized to contain at least **50% EGCG**, with a suggested dosage of **250-500 mg per day**.

Resveratrol is a polyphenol found in the skin of red grapes, berries, and peanuts. It's well-regarded for its anti-aging properties and ability to improve heart health and longevity. For those looking to add resveratrol to their diet, **trans-resveratrol supplements** are the most bioavailable form. The recommended dosage ranges from **100-500 mg per day**. As with any supplement, it's critical to choose products that are third-party tested for quality and potency.

Materials Needed:
- Natural astaxanthin supplements (4-12 mg)
- Organic loose-leaf green tea or green tea extract (250-500 mg standardized to 50% EGCG)
- Trans-resveratrol supplements (100-500 mg)
- A reliable source for purchasing high-quality supplements

Preparation and Application Steps:
1. **Astaxanthin**: Take one capsule of astaxanthin daily, preferably with a meal containing fat, as it's fat-soluble and this enhances absorption.
2. **Green Tea**: Brew 1 teaspoon of loose-leaf green tea in 8 ounces of hot water for 3-5 minutes. Enjoy 2-3 cups throughout the day. If using an extract, follow the dosage instructions on the product label.
3. **Resveratrol**: Consume resveratrol supplement as directed, ideally with meals to improve absorption due to its fat-soluble nature.

Safety Considerations:
- Always consult with a healthcare provider before beginning any new supplement, especially if you have existing health conditions or are taking medications.
- Start with the lower end of the recommended dosages and monitor your body's response before gradually increasing.
- Ensure all supplements are stored properly, away from direct sunlight and moisture, to maintain their potency.
- Be aware of potential interactions between these supplements and medications, particularly blood thinners and immune-suppressing drugs.

Incorporating these antioxidants into your daily routine can be a powerful step towards enhancing longevity and overall well-being. By selecting high-quality supplements and following the recommended dosages and safety guidelines, you can maximize the benefits of these potent herbal antioxidants.

Adaptogenic Herbs for Stress and Aging

Adaptogenic herbs have gained recognition for their unique ability to **enhance the body's resistance to stress** and support healthy aging. Among these, **Ashwagandha**, **Rhodiola Rosea**, and **Holy Basil** stand out for their efficacy and safety profile. These herbs work by modulating the body's stress response systems, providing support for both mental and physical aspects of aging.

Ashwagandha (Withania somnifera), also known as Indian ginseng, is revered for its ability to reduce cortisol levels, combat stress, and improve energy levels. For optimal results, consider a daily dosage of **300-500 mg** of a high-concentration, full-spectrum extract. It's crucial to select a product standardized to contain at least **5% withanolides**, the active compounds responsible for its therapeutic effects.

Materials Needed:
- Ashwagandha extract capsules, standardized to 5% withanolides
- A daily planner or reminder system to maintain consistency in supplementation

Preparation and Application Steps:
1. Start with **300 mg of Ashwagandha extract** daily, taken with meals to enhance absorption. If your product comes in higher dosages, adjust accordingly by taking fewer capsules.
2. Monitor your body's response over a period of 2-4 weeks, gradually increasing the dosage to 500 mg if needed and well-tolerated.
3. Consistency is key. Set reminders to take the supplement at the same time each day to establish a routine and maximize its stress-reducing benefits.

Rhodiola Rosea is another powerful adaptogen known for its fatigue-reducing and cognitive-enhancing properties. When selecting a Rhodiola supplement, aim for one that provides **3% rosavins and 1% salidroside**, reflecting the natural ratio of these compounds in the plant.

Materials Needed:
- Rhodiola Rosea extract, standardized to 3% rosavins and 1% salidroside
- A journal to note any changes in energy levels, cognitive function, or stress levels

Preparation and Application Steps:
1. Begin with a dose of **100 mg of Rhodiola Rosea extract** in the morning, preferably 30 minutes before breakfast.
2. Observe your body's reaction for one week, noting any improvements in energy, mood, or mental clarity.
3. If well-tolerated, increase the dosage to 200 mg daily, split into two doses taken before breakfast and lunch to avoid potential sleep disturbances.

Holy Basil (Ocimum sanctum), or Tulsi, is celebrated in Ayurvedic medicine for its adaptogenic and anti-anxiety effects. For daily supplementation, dried leaf powder, teas, or extracts can be used, with a general recommendation of **300-600 mg** of extract per day.

Materials Needed:
- Holy Basil leaf powder or extract
- Tea infuser or capsule machine if using loose powder

Preparation and Application Steps:

1. For tea, steep 1 teaspoon of Holy Basil leaf powder in hot water for 5-10 minutes. Drink 1-2 cups daily to enjoy its stress-relieving benefits.
2. If using an extract, start with 300 mg daily, divided into two doses to be taken with meals.
3. Adjust the dosage based on your response, up to a maximum of 600 mg per day, ensuring no adverse effects are experienced.

Safety Considerations:
- While adaptogenic herbs are generally safe, individual reactions can vary. Start with lower dosages and gradually adjust.
- Pregnant or breastfeeding women should avoid using these herbs due to limited research on their safety in these populations.
- Consult with a healthcare provider before beginning any new supplement regimen, especially if you have existing health conditions or are taking other medications.

Incorporating adaptogenic herbs into your daily routine can be a strategic approach to managing stress and supporting healthy aging. By carefully selecting high-quality supplements and adhering to the recommended dosages and safety guidelines, you can leverage the natural power of these herbs to enhance your resilience to stress and promote overall well-being.

Natural Joint and Bone Support

For those seeking **natural joint and bone support**, focusing on **Calcium**, **Magnesium**, **Vitamin D**, and **Omega-3 fatty acids** is crucial. These nutrients play a pivotal role in maintaining bone density and joint health, which are essential for aging gracefully. Incorporating foods rich in these nutrients along with specific supplements can significantly impact your overall bone and joint well-being.

Calcium is fundamental for bone health. The recommended daily intake for adults is 1,000 mg, which increases to 1,200 mg for women over 50 and men over 70. To ensure adequate calcium intake, include dairy products like milk, cheese, and yogurt in your diet. For those who are dairy-intolerant or vegan, options like fortified plant milks, kale, and almonds are excellent sources. If dietary sources are insufficient, consider a calcium supplement, but choose one that's easily absorbable, such as calcium citrate or calcium carbonate, taking it with meals to enhance absorption.

Magnesium works in tandem with calcium by contributing to the structural development of bones and is necessary for the synthesis of DNA and RNA. Adults should aim for 400-420 mg (men) and 310-320 mg (women) daily. Magnesium-rich foods include leafy green vegetables, nuts, seeds, and whole grains. If opting for a supplement, magnesium glycinate is a good choice due to its high bioavailability and lower likelihood of causing digestive discomfort.

Vitamin D is critical for calcium absorption and bone health. The recommended daily intake is 600 IU for adults up to age 70 and 800 IU for those older. Sunlight is a natural source of Vitamin D, but with limited exposure, especially in winter months, supplementation may be necessary. Vitamin D3 supplements are preferred for their effectiveness in raising and maintaining adequate levels in the body.

Omega-3 fatty acids, found in fish oil, have anti-inflammatory properties that can alleviate joint pain and stiffness. For joint health, a daily intake of 250-500 mg of EPA and DHA, the active forms of omega-3, is recommended. While fatty fish like salmon, mackerel, and sardines are the best sources, a high-quality fish oil supplement can also be beneficial, especially for those who do not consume fish regularly.

Materials Needed:
- Calcium supplement (citrate or carbonate)
- Magnesium glycinate supplement
- Vitamin D3 supplement
- Fish oil supplement rich in EPA and DHA
- Grocery list including dairy or fortified plant milks, leafy greens, nuts, seeds, and fatty fish

Preparation and Application Steps:
1. **Dietary Integration**: Plan weekly meals to include calcium and magnesium-rich foods. Incorporate fatty fish into your diet 2-3 times per week for omega-3s.
2. **Supplementation**: If sunlight exposure is limited, take a Vitamin D3 supplement with the largest meal of the day to enhance absorption. For calcium and magnesium, consider your dietary intake and supplement as needed, ideally with meals. Take fish oil supplements with meals to improve absorption and minimize any potential aftertaste.
3. **Monitoring and Adjustment**: Keep a journal of your dietary intake and supplement usage to monitor your nutrient levels. Adjust as necessary based on how your body responds, aiming for the recommended daily intake through a combination of diet and supplements.
4. **Consultation**: Before starting any new supplement regimen, consult with a healthcare provider, especially if you have existing health conditions or are taking medications.

Incorporating these nutrients into your daily routine can support joint and bone health, contributing to a more active and pain-free lifestyle as you age. By carefully selecting high-quality supplements and prioritizing nutrient-rich foods, you can effectively support your body's natural processes and enhance your overall well-being.

Herbs for Arthritis and Inflammation

For individuals seeking natural remedies to alleviate arthritis and inflammation, incorporating specific herbs into their daily regimen can offer significant relief. These herbs, known for their anti-inflammatory and pain-relieving properties, can be used in various forms such as teas, tinctures, capsules, or topical applications. Here, we detail the use of **Boswellia Serrata**, **Ginger**, and **Turmeric** for managing arthritis and inflammation effectively.

Boswellia Serrata, also known as Indian frankincense, contains active compounds called boswellic acids that block the production of pro-inflammatory enzymes. For optimal benefits, look for **Boswellia supplements standardized to contain at least 65% boswellic acids**. The recommended dosage is **300-500 mg** taken two to three times daily with meals to enhance absorption. When shopping for Boswellia, ensure the product is third-party tested to verify its purity and potency.

Materials Needed:
- Boswellia Serrata supplements (standardized to 65% boswellic acids)
- A pill organizer to manage dosages throughout the day

Preparation and Application Steps:
1. Begin with a **300 mg dose of Boswellia**, three times a day with meals. This can help maintain consistent levels of the herb in your body.
2. After two weeks, assess your body's response. If necessary, and well-tolerated, increase the dosage to 500 mg three times a day to maximize anti-inflammatory effects.
3. Maintain a log of your dosage and any changes in symptoms to discuss with your healthcare provider, ensuring the supplement's efficacy and safety.

Ginger is another powerful herb with pronounced anti-inflammatory and analgesic properties, attributed to its compounds gingerols and shogaols. To incorporate ginger for arthritis relief, you can use fresh ginger root in cooking, or take a **ginger supplement**. The recommended dosage for ginger supplements is **100-200 mg** up to three times daily. Ensure the supplement is standardized to contain gingerols for maximum benefit.

Materials Needed:
- Fresh ginger root or ginger supplements (standardized to contain gingerols)
- A kitchen grater if using fresh ginger

Preparation and Application Steps:
1. For fresh ginger, grate approximately one tablespoon and add it to meals or steep in hot water to make ginger tea. Consume two to three times daily.
2. If using a supplement, start with 100 mg three times a day with meals. Adjust the dosage based on your response and tolerance, not exceeding 600 mg daily.
3. Keep a record of your intake and any symptom relief or side effects to gauge effectiveness and adjust as needed.

Turmeric, celebrated for its curcumin content, offers significant anti-inflammatory benefits. To enhance curcumin absorption, combine **turmeric with black pepper** (piperine). The recommended dosage for turmeric supplements is **500-2,000 mg** of curcumin per day, divided into two doses. Look for supplements that contain piperine or are formulated for enhanced absorption.

Materials Needed:

- Turmeric supplements containing curcumin, ideally with piperine or formulated for enhanced absorption
- Measuring spoons for accurate dosing if using turmeric powder

Preparation and Application Steps:

1. If using turmeric powder, incorporate one to two teaspoons into your diet daily, combined with a pinch of black pepper to enhance absorption. This can be added to smoothies, soups, or rice dishes.
2. For supplements, start with a 500 mg dose twice daily, with meals. Monitor your body's response, and if well-tolerated, you may increase the dosage, aiming for a total of 2,000 mg of curcumin per day.
3. Document your supplement intake and observe any changes in inflammation or pain levels to fine-tune your regimen.

Safety Considerations:

- While these herbs are generally considered safe, it's crucial to start with lower dosages and gradually increase to assess tolerance.
- Pregnant or nursing women, individuals with existing health conditions, or those on medication should consult a healthcare provider before starting any new supplement.
- Monitor for any adverse reactions, such as digestive upset, and adjust dosages accordingly or discontinue use.

By integrating **Boswellia Serrata**, **Ginger**, and **Turmeric** into your daily routine, you can harness their natural anti-inflammatory and analgesic properties to support joint health and reduce inflammation. Remember to choose high-quality supplements, follow recommended dosages, and consult with a healthcare provider to tailor these remedies to your specific needs.

Chapter 8: Mental and Emotional Well-being

Herbs for Anxiety and Depression

Anxiety and depression are common mental health concerns that can significantly impact daily life. While conventional treatments are available, many individuals seek natural remedies for relief. Herbs have been used for centuries to alleviate symptoms of anxiety and depression, offering a holistic approach to mental well-being. It's essential to understand how specific herbs can be utilized effectively and safely to support emotional health.

St. John's Wort is widely recognized for its antidepressant properties. It contains active compounds such as hypericin and hyperforin, which are thought to influence neurotransmitters in the brain related to mood regulation. For those considering St. John's Wort, a standard dosage is 300 mg of an extract standardized to 0.3% hypericin or 3-5% hyperforin, taken three times daily. It's crucial to note that St. John's Wort can interact with a variety of medications, including birth control pills, antidepressants, and blood thinners, so consulting with a healthcare provider before starting is advised.

Materials Needed:
- St. John's Wort extract (standardized to 0.3% hypericin or 3-5% hyperforin)
- A journal to track mood changes and potential side effects

Preparation and Application Steps:
1. Begin with the lower end of the recommended dosage, taking one 300 mg capsule with meals to enhance absorption and reduce the risk of stomach upset.
2. Monitor your response closely, noting any changes in mood, energy levels, or side effects in a journal. This documentation can be invaluable for adjusting dosages or assessing the effectiveness of the treatment.
3. Consistency is key when using St. John's Wort. Maintain a regular dosing schedule, and allow several weeks to observe significant effects, as the full benefits may take time to manifest.

Lavender is renowned for its calming and sedative effects, making it an excellent choice for those dealing with anxiety. Lavender can be used in various forms, including essential oils, teas, and capsules. For anxiety relief, lavender oil aromatherapy has been shown to reduce symptoms effectively. A few drops of lavender essential oil can be added to a diffuser or inhaled directly from the bottle during moments of stress.

Materials Needed:
- Lavender essential oil

- A diffuser for aromatherapy or a small cloth for inhalation

Preparation and Application Steps:

1. For aromatherapy, add 5-10 drops of lavender essential oil to a diffuser filled with water. Place the diffuser in a room where you spend a lot of time, such as a bedroom or office, to provide continuous exposure to the calming scent.
2. If direct inhalation is preferred, place 2-3 drops of lavender oil on a small cloth or handkerchief. Hold it near your nose and take deep, slow breaths for several minutes. This method can be particularly effective for acute anxiety relief.
3. Incorporate lavender into your evening routine to promote relaxation and improve sleep quality. A few drops of lavender oil can be added to a warm bath or applied to the pillow before bedtime.

Safety Considerations:

- While lavender is generally safe, it's important to conduct a patch test before topical application to rule out any allergic reactions.
- Pregnant or nursing women should consult a healthcare provider before using lavender, especially in medicinal amounts.
- Essential oils are potent, and direct contact with the skin should be avoided unless diluted with a carrier oil.

By integrating St. John's Wort and Lavender into your mental health regimen, you can harness their natural properties to combat anxiety and depression. Remember, natural remedies can complement but not replace conventional treatments, so it's critical to communicate with a healthcare professional about your mental health strategy.

Passionflower has been traditionally used to alleviate symptoms of anxiety and insomnia, acting as a natural sedative. The compounds in passionflower, including flavonoids and alkaloids, are believed to interact with neurotransmitter receptors in the brain to promote relaxation. For managing anxiety, the recommended dosage of passionflower extract is 400-800 mg daily, divided into two or three doses. It can also be consumed as tea; steep 1 teaspoon of dried passionflower in boiling water for 10 minutes and drink this infusion 1-2 times daily.

Materials Needed:

- Passionflower extract or dried passionflower for tea
- A teapot or cup for brewing tea

Preparation and Application Steps:

1. If using passionflower extract, start with a 200 mg dose twice daily to assess tolerance. Gradually increase to 400 mg twice daily if needed, based on your response and as tolerated.

2. For tea, place 1 teaspoon of dried passionflower in a cup of boiling water and allow it to steep for 10 minutes. Strain the tea and enjoy it before bedtime or during moments of heightened anxiety.
3. Keep track of your dosage and any changes in anxiety levels or sleep quality to adjust the amount consumed as necessary.

Lemon Balm, another herb known for its calming effects, can help reduce anxiety and improve mood. The active compounds in lemon balm, including rosmarinic acid, have been shown to increase the availability of neurotransmitters in the brain that regulate mood. Lemon balm can be taken as a tea, extract, or in capsule form. A typical dosage for anxiety relief is 300-600 mg of lemon balm extract daily, or 1-2 cups of lemon balm tea.

Materials Needed:
- Lemon balm extract, dried leaves for tea, or capsules
- A teapot or cup for brewing tea

Preparation and Application Steps:
1. To prepare lemon balm tea, steep 1-2 teaspoons of dried lemon balm leaves in boiling water for 5-10 minutes. Drink this tea 1-2 times daily, especially in the evening to promote relaxation.
2. If opting for lemon balm extract or capsules, begin with the lower dosage of 300 mg per day. Observe your body's response over a week, then adjust the dosage up to 600 mg if needed and tolerated.
3. Document your intake and note any improvements in anxiety symptoms or overall mood to help gauge the effectiveness of lemon balm in your regimen.

Safety Considerations:
- Passionflower and lemon balm are generally considered safe for most adults, but it's important to start with lower doses to assess individual tolerance.
- Individuals taking sedatives or medications for insomnia should consult with a healthcare provider before using passionflower or lemon balm, as they may enhance the effects of these drugs.
- As with any supplement, pregnant or nursing women should seek medical advice before incorporating passionflower or lemon balm into their routine.

Incorporating herbs like St. John's Wort, Lavender, Passionflower, and Lemon Balm into your daily routine offers a natural approach to managing anxiety and depression. Each herb provides unique benefits, and when used responsibly under the guidance of a healthcare provider, can contribute to improved mental and emotional well-being. Always consider your personal health history and potential interactions with other medications when exploring herbal remedies for anxiety and depression.

Herbs for Anxiety and Depression

Ashwagandha has gained recognition for its ability to reduce stress and anxiety. This adaptogenic herb works by moderating the stress response, potentially lowering cortisol levels. For those looking to incorporate Ashwagandha into their regimen, the recommended starting dosage is **300 mg**, taken twice daily. The extract should be standardized to contain at least 5% withanolides, which are the active compounds. When selecting Ashwagandha supplements, ensure they are from a reputable source and have been third-party tested for purity and potency.

Materials Needed:
- Ashwagandha extract capsules, standardized to 5% withanolides
- A daily planner or app to track dosage times and effects

Preparation and Application Steps:
1. Start with **300 mg of Ashwagandha extract** in the morning, preferably with breakfast to enhance absorption.
2. Take another **300 mg dose** in the evening with dinner to maintain consistent levels of the herb in your system.
3. Note any changes in stress levels, sleep quality, and overall well-being in a daily planner or app to monitor the herb's effectiveness over time.

Chamomile is well-known for its calming properties, making it an excellent choice for those dealing with anxiety and stress. It can be consumed as tea or taken in capsule form. For tea, steep **2-3 teaspoons of dried chamomile flowers** in hot water for 10 minutes. Drink 1-2 cups in the evening or whenever you need to calm your nerves. If you prefer capsules, look for products standardized to contain **1.2% apigenin**, the active compound, and follow the manufacturer's recommended dosage.

Materials Needed:
- Dried chamomile flowers or chamomile capsules standardized to 1.2% apigenin
- Teapot or cup for brewing tea

Preparation and Application Steps:
1. For chamomile tea, place **2-3 teaspoons of dried flowers** in a cup of boiling water. Allow it to steep for 10 minutes before straining.
2. Consume **1-2 cups of chamomile tea** in the evening to promote relaxation and improve sleep quality.
3. If using capsules, take as directed by the product label, usually once or twice daily, to support anxiety reduction.

Valerian Root has been traditionally used to improve sleep and reduce anxiety. Its sedative effects can be attributed to the valerenic acid it contains. To use valerian root for anxiety, the recommended dosage in capsule form is **300 to 600 mg**, taken 30 minutes to 2 hours before bedtime. Ensure the supplement is standardized to contain **0.8% valerenic acid** for optimal effectiveness.

Materials Needed:
- Valerian root capsules standardized to 0.8% valerenic acid
- A journal to track sleep patterns and anxiety levels

Preparation and Application Steps:
1. Begin with a **300 mg dose of valerian root** in the evening, adjusting the timing based on your bedtime to find what works best for you.
2. Gradually increase the dosage to **600 mg** if needed, based on your response and the severity of your anxiety.
3. Keep a journal to document any changes in your sleep quality and anxiety levels, which can help in determining the most effective dose for you.

Safety Considerations:
- While these herbs are generally considered safe, it's important to start with the recommended dosages and gradually adjust based on your body's response.
- Pregnant or nursing women should avoid these herbs or consult a healthcare provider before use.
- Individuals with existing health conditions or those taking medications should consult a healthcare provider to avoid potential interactions.
- Monitor for any adverse reactions and consult a healthcare provider if you experience any concerning symptoms.

Incorporating Ashwagandha, Chamomile, and Valerian Root into your daily routine can offer a natural approach to managing anxiety and depression. These herbs have been used for centuries and are backed by modern research supporting their efficacy in improving mental and emotional well-being. By following the recommended dosages and preparation steps, and considering the safety considerations, you can safely explore these natural remedies as part of your overall strategy for reducing anxiety and enhancing your mood.

Mood-Lifting Teas and Tinctures

Building on the foundation of utilizing herbs for mental and emotional well-being, mood-lifting teas and tinctures present a potent avenue for enhancing mood and combating the symptoms of anxiety and depression. The preparation of these remedies involves precise measurements and specific techniques to ensure their efficacy and safety. When crafting mood-lifting teas and tinctures, it is crucial to select high-quality, organic herbs known for their mood-enhancing properties. Among these, **Rhodiola Rosea**, **Holy Basil**, and **Saffron** stand out for their scientifically supported benefits in improving mood and mental clarity.

Rhodiola Rosea, often referred to as the 'golden root', is a remarkable adaptogen that aids in increasing resistance to stress while boosting energy levels and mood. To prepare a Rhodiola tincture, one must:

1. Obtain **Rhodiola Rosea root**, either in dried form or freshly harvested. If using fresh root, chop it finely to increase the surface area for extraction.
2. Measure approximately **1 part Rhodiola to 5 parts alcohol** (vodka or grain alcohol) for the tincture. For those preferring a non-alcoholic version, glycerin can be used, though the extraction might be less potent.
3. Combine the Rhodiola and alcohol in a glass jar, ensuring the root is completely submerged. Seal the jar tightly and store it in a cool, dark place for 4 to 6 weeks, shaking it gently every few days to facilitate extraction.
4. After the steeping period, strain the mixture through a fine mesh strainer or cheesecloth, squeezing out as much liquid as possible. Transfer the tincture to a clean, dark glass dropper bottle for easy use.
5. The recommended dosage starts at **20-30 drops** taken in water or juice, once to twice daily. It is essential to observe how your body responds and adjust the dosage accordingly.

Holy Basil, also known as Tulsi, is revered for its stress-reducing and mood-enhancing properties. To make a Holy Basil tea:

1. Start with **2 teaspoons of dried Holy Basil leaves** per cup of boiling water. For those with access to fresh leaves, a handful can be used to create a more potent infusion.
2. Add the Holy Basil to a teapot or cup and pour boiling water over the leaves. Cover and allow it to steep for **5-10 minutes**. The longer it steeps, the stronger the tea will be.
3. Strain the leaves from the tea and serve hot. For added flavor and benefits, a teaspoon of honey or lemon can be added. This tea can be consumed **1-2 times daily** to help elevate mood and reduce stress.

Saffron, known for its vibrant color and distinctive flavor, has been shown to have mood-enhancing effects comparable to some antidepressants. Creating a saffron tincture involves:

1. Acquiring high-quality **saffron threads**; about **1 gram** will suffice for a small batch of tincture.
2. Place the saffron threads in a glass jar and cover with **1 cup of alcohol** (vodka or grain alcohol is preferred for its neutral flavor).
3. Seal the jar and store it in a dark, cool place, allowing the saffron to infuse for at least 2 weeks. Shake the jar every couple of days to ensure even extraction.
4. After the infusion period, strain the tincture into a dark glass bottle fitted with a dropper for ease of dosage.
5. Saffron tincture can be used by adding **5-10 drops** to water or tea and consumed once daily. As with any herbal remedy, it's crucial to monitor your body's response and adjust the dosage as needed.

When incorporating these mood-lifting teas and tinctures into your regimen, it's vital to consider any potential interactions with medications or underlying health conditions. Consulting with a healthcare provider before starting any new herbal treatment is recommended, especially for those with existing medical concerns or those who are pregnant or breastfeeding. Additionally, maintaining a record of your herbal intake, along with any changes in mood and overall well-being, can be beneficial in tracking the effectiveness of these natural remedies and making necessary adjustments. Through careful selection and preparation of these mood-lifting herbs, individuals can harness their natural properties to support mental and emotional health, contributing to a holistic approach to well-being.

Cognitive Function and Memory

Ginkgo Biloba is renowned for its capacity to enhance cognitive function and memory. This ancient herb acts by improving blood flow to the brain, thereby supporting brain health and cognitive processes. For those looking to incorporate Ginkgo Biloba into their cognitive health regimen, the recommended dosage is **120 to 240 mg** of a standardized extract, divided into two or three doses throughout the day. It is crucial to select products standardized to contain 24% flavone glycosides and 6% terpene lactones, the active compounds responsible for Ginkgo's cognitive benefits.

Materials Needed:
- Ginkgo Biloba extract, standardized to 24% flavone glycosides and 6% terpene lactones
- A pill organizer to manage multiple daily doses

Preparation and Application Steps:
1. Begin with a **120 mg dose** of Ginkgo Biloba extract in the morning, taken with breakfast to enhance absorption.
2. Take a second dose, either **120 mg** at noon with lunch or **60 mg** at noon and another **60 mg** in the late afternoon, to maintain consistent levels of the herb in your system.
3. Consistently use Ginkgo Biloba for at least **4-6 weeks** before evaluating its impact on your cognitive function and memory. This timeframe allows the herb to accumulate in your system and exert its beneficial effects.

Lion's Mane Mushroom is another powerful natural remedy for cognitive enhancement. This unique mushroom supports the growth of nerve growth factors, which are essential for brain health. To incorporate Lion's Mane into your diet, look for a high-quality extract or powder. The recommended dosage for cognitive benefits is **500 to 1000 mg** of the extract, taken twice daily.

Materials Needed:
- Lion's Mane Mushroom extract or powder
- Measuring spoon for accurate dosage

Preparation and Application Steps:
1. If using Lion's Mane extract, take **500 mg** in the morning with breakfast.
2. Take another **500 mg** dose in the evening with dinner.
3. For those using powder form, it can be mixed into smoothies, coffee, or tea. Ensure the daily intake totals **1000 to 2000 mg**.

Bacopa Monnieri, commonly known as Brahmi, is a traditional Ayurvedic herb used for improving memory and cognitive function. It works by enhancing neurotransmitter function and protecting brain cells from oxidative stress. The optimal dosage of Bacopa Monnieri for cognitive enhancement is **300 mg** of an extract standardized to contain at least 55% bacosides, taken once daily.

Materials Needed:
- Bacopa Monnieri extract, standardized to at least 55% bacosides
- A daily planner to track dosage and cognitive changes

Preparation and Application Steps:
1. Take **300 mg** of Bacopa Monnieri extract in the morning, preferably with food to minimize potential gastrointestinal discomfort.
2. Consistent daily intake is crucial, as the cognitive benefits of Bacopa Monnieri build over time. Evaluate its effects on memory and cognitive function after **8-12 weeks**.

Safety Considerations:
- When starting any new supplement, particularly those aimed at enhancing cognitive function, it is essential to monitor for any adverse reactions or side effects.
- Pregnant or nursing women, individuals with existing health conditions, or those on medication should consult a healthcare provider before starting any new supplement regimen.
- Ginkgo Biloba may interact with blood-thinning medications. It is crucial to consult with a healthcare provider if you are taking any such medications.
- Consistency in taking these supplements as directed is key to observing significant improvements in cognitive function and memory.

Nootropic Herbs for Brain Health

Expanding upon the foundation of cognitive enhancement through natural means, Phosphatidylserine stands out as a critical compound for brain health. This phospholipid is integral to the structure of cell membranes and plays a pivotal role in maintaining cognitive functions, including memory, concentration, and the overall health of brain cells. For those considering Phosphatidylserine supplementation, it is recommended to start with a dosage of 100 mg taken three times a day. This supplement is derived either from soy or sunflower lecithin, making it important for consumers to choose a product based on their dietary preferences or restrictions. Ensuring the supplement is from a reputable manufacturer that provides third-party testing for purity and potency can offer additional assurance of its quality.

Materials needed for incorporating Phosphatidylserine into a cognitive health regimen include Phosphatidylserine supplements clearly labeled with the source (soy or sunflower) and standardized to contain at least 20% phosphatidylserine. A daily planner or digital app can be beneficial for tracking dosage times and noting any changes in cognitive function or mood, aiding individuals in monitoring the supplement's effectiveness over time.

Preparation and application steps involve taking one 100 mg capsule of Phosphatidylserine with meals in the morning, midday, and evening to optimize absorption and ensure a consistent level of the compound in the body. Observing the body's response over a period of 4-6 weeks is crucial, as this timeframe allows for an accurate assessment of the supplement's impact on cognitive functions. Adjustments to the dosage should be made in consultation with a healthcare provider, especially if other medications are being taken or if there are pre-existing health conditions.

Another noteworthy herb for enhancing cognitive function is Huperzine A, derived from the Chinese club moss, Huperzia serrata. Huperzine A acts as a cholinesterase inhibitor, which means it helps increase levels of neurotransmitters in the brain. This action supports memory, learning capabilities, and overall brain function. The recommended starting dosage for Huperzine A is 50 mcg taken twice daily. Given its potent effects, it is essential to begin with the lowest possible dose and gradually adjust based on personal tolerance and response.

Materials needed include Huperzine A supplements, preferably those that have been third-party tested for purity and contain a standardized amount of the active ingredient. As with Phosphatidylserine, maintaining a log of dosage, timing, and any cognitive changes can help users gauge the effectiveness of Huperzine A in their cognitive enhancement efforts.

Preparation and application steps for Huperzine A involve taking one 50 mcg capsule in the morning and another in the early afternoon, ideally with food to mitigate any potential gastrointestinal discomfort. Monitoring cognitive improvements or side effects daily provides valuable feedback for adjusting the dosage as needed. It's also advisable to cycle Huperzine A, taking it for a period followed by a break, to prevent tolerance build-up and ensure its long-term efficacy.

Safety considerations for both Phosphatidylserine and Huperzine A include awareness of potential interactions with medications, particularly those affecting the brain and nervous system. Pregnant or nursing women should avoid these supplements due to the lack of extensive research on their safety in these populations. Individuals should consult with a healthcare provider to ensure these nootropic supplements are appropriate for their health profile and to avoid adverse interactions with existing treatments.

By integrating Phosphatidylserine and Huperzine A into a regimen focused on cognitive health, individuals can leverage the neuroprotective and cognitive-enhancing properties of these compounds. Careful adherence to recommended dosages, vigilant monitoring of effects, and consultation with healthcare professionals can maximize the benefits of these nootropic herbs while minimizing potential risks, contributing to the overarching goal of improved brain health and enhanced cognitive function.

Chapter 9: Herbal Skincare and Beauty

In the realm of herbal skincare and beauty, the focus on natural, plant-based ingredients marks a return to ancient practices that honor the body's inherent connection to the earth. The use of herbs in skincare is not only about enhancing beauty but also about promoting skin health through the potent properties of plants. For individuals seeking to integrate herbal remedies into their skincare routine, understanding the specific benefits of various herbs and how to apply them effectively is crucial.

Aloe Vera is renowned for its soothing, hydrating properties, making it an essential ingredient in natural skincare formulations. To harness the benefits of Aloe Vera, one can extract the gel directly from the plant's leaves. This gel can be applied topically to moisturize the skin, treat burns, and reduce inflammation. For a simple Aloe Vera face mask, mix 2 tablespoons of fresh Aloe Vera gel with 1 teaspoon of honey and apply to the face for 15-20 minutes before rinsing with warm water. This mask not only hydrates but also provides antibacterial benefits, thanks to the honey.

Calendula, with its anti-inflammatory and healing properties, is another cornerstone of herbal skincare. Infused oils are a popular way to incorporate Calendula into beauty routines. To create a Calendula oil infusion, fill a jar with dried Calendula flowers and cover with a carrier oil such as jojoba or almond oil. Seal the jar and place it in a warm, sunny spot for 4-6 weeks, shaking it occasionally. The resulting oil can be applied directly to the skin to soothe irritations, heal minor cuts, and improve overall skin texture.

Green Tea is packed with antioxidants and can be used in various skincare applications to protect against environmental damage and aging. A simple way to include Green Tea in skincare is by brewing a strong cup of tea, allowing it to cool, and then using it as a facial toner. This toner can be applied with a cotton ball after cleansing to tighten pores, reduce redness, and provide an antioxidant boost.

Lavender is not only cherished for its calming aroma but also for its ability to soothe the skin. Lavender hydrosol, a by-product of the distillation process used to extract essential oils, serves as a gentle facial toner suitable for all skin types. It can calm skin irritations, reduce redness, and promote a sense of relaxation. To use, spray Lavender hydrosol onto the face after cleansing, or add it to homemade beauty formulations for its therapeutic benefits.

For those interested in exfoliation, **Oatmeal** serves as a gentle, natural exfoliant suitable for even the most sensitive skin. A homemade oatmeal scrub can be made by grinding whole oats in a food processor and mixing them with honey and a small amount of water to form a paste. Applied in gentle circular motions, this scrub can remove dead skin cells without stripping the skin of its natural oils.

Incorporating these herbal ingredients into a skincare routine not only promotes skin health but also aligns with a holistic approach to wellness that values natural, sustainable practices. As we delve deeper into the world of herbal skincare and beauty, it becomes evident that the power of plants can be effectively harnessed to not only enhance our external appearance but also to support the body's natural healing processes.

Rosehip Seed Oil emerges as a champion for its remarkable skin rejuvenating and hydrating properties. Rich in essential fatty acids and vitamins A and C, Rosehip Seed Oil can be applied directly to the skin to help reduce the appearance of scars, fine lines, and hyperpigmentation. For an effective nightly serum, mix together 5 drops of Rosehip Seed Oil, 2 drops of Frankincense essential oil, and 3 drops of Lavender essential oil. This blend not only moisturizes but also harnesses the anti-aging and soothing properties of the essential oils.

Witch Hazel, known for its astringent qualities, is invaluable for those with oily or acne-prone skin. It can be used as a natural toner to remove excess oil, tighten pores, and reduce inflammation. To enhance its benefits, combine Witch Hazel with tea tree oil—a powerful antibacterial agent—to create a homemade acne treatment solution. Simply mix 1 cup of Witch Hazel with 10 drops of tea tree oil in a clean bottle. Apply with a cotton pad after cleansing to help keep acne at bay.

Chamomile is celebrated for its calming and anti-inflammatory effects on the skin. A Chamomile tea facial steam is an excellent way to harness these benefits, helping to soothe and cleanse the skin. Boil a pot of water and add 2 tablespoons of dried Chamomile flowers, allowing them to steep for 5 minutes. Then, with a towel over your head, gently lean over the pot at a safe distance, letting the steam envelop your face for about 10 minutes. This method not only calms the skin but also opens the pores for deeper cleansing.

Sea Buckthorn Oil is packed with antioxidants, vitamins, and essential fatty acids, making it a powerful ally for skin health. Its high concentration of Vitamin C and E promotes skin hydration, elasticity, and regeneration. For a rejuvenating face oil, blend 3 drops of Sea Buckthorn Oil with 5 drops of Argan oil and 2 drops of Rose essential oil. Apply a few drops of this mixture to the face before bed to nourish the skin overnight.

Neem Oil has a long history of use in traditional medicine for its antiseptic, anti-inflammatory, and moisturizing properties. It is particularly beneficial for skin conditions like eczema, psoriasis, and acne. Create a healing balm by melting 2 tablespoons of Shea butter, then stirring in 10 drops of Neem Oil and 5 drops of Lavender essential oil until well combined. Once cooled, apply to affected areas to soothe irritation and promote healing.

In exploring these diverse herbal ingredients and their applications, it's clear that nature provides a vast array of options for nurturing and maintaining healthy skin. By selecting the right herbs and natural substances, tailored to individual skin needs and concerns, one can create a personalized skincare regimen that supports skin health and beauty from the inside out. Through the thoughtful incorporation of these herbal remedies, we embrace a more sustainable, effective approach to skincare that honors the wisdom of nature and our bodies' natural rhythms.

Natural Facial Care

Turmeric is a potent anti-inflammatory and antioxidant herb, widely recognized for its skin brightening and healing properties. To create a turmeric face mask, mix 1 teaspoon of turmeric powder with 2 teaspoons of yogurt and a few drops of honey until a smooth paste is formed. Apply this mixture to clean, dry skin, leaving it on for 15-20 minutes before rinsing with lukewarm water. This mask can help reduce acne scars and inflammation, leaving the skin glowing and smooth. It's important to use organic turmeric powder to avoid any additives or dyes that could irritate the skin. For those with lighter skin tones, be cautious as turmeric can temporarily stain the skin yellow; a patch test is recommended.

Tea Tree Oil is renowned for its antibacterial and anti-inflammatory qualities, making it an excellent choice for treating acne and oily skin types. To utilize tea tree oil in your skincare routine, add 2-3 drops to a tablespoon of witch hazel and apply it directly to blemishes using a cotton swab. This solution can be used once daily to help reduce redness and prevent acne breakouts. Ensure you're using 100% pure tea tree oil and dilute it appropriately to avoid skin irritation.

Cucumber is not only hydrating but also possesses soothing properties that are beneficial for the skin, especially for calming irritated or sunburned skin. For a refreshing cucumber toner, blend one fresh cucumber with a half cup of water until smooth. Strain the mixture to extract the juice, then apply it to the face with a cotton ball or spray bottle. Store the remaining toner in the refrigerator for up to one week. The cooling effect of cucumber helps soothe the skin, while its natural astringent properties tighten pores.

Rose Water has been used for centuries as a facial toner due to its ability to balance the skin's pH, reduce redness, and hydrate. For daily use, simply soak a cotton pad with rose water and gently apply it to your face after cleansing. This step can help prep your skin for moisturizers and serums, enhancing their absorption and efficacy. Opt for pure, organic rose water to ensure your skin receives the full benefits without any harmful additives.

Jojoba Oil is a lightweight, non-comedogenic oil that closely mimics the skin's natural sebum, making it an excellent moisturizer for all skin types, including oily and acne-prone skin. To incorporate jojoba oil into your skincare routine, apply a few drops to your face after cleansing and toning, gently massaging it into your skin. Jojoba oil can also be used as a carrier oil for diluting essential oils or as a base for homemade skincare formulations. Its anti-inflammatory properties help soothe the skin, while its moisturizing benefits prevent dryness and promote a healthy skin barrier.

Green Clay offers detoxifying properties, making it ideal for deep cleansing and refining pores. For an effective green clay mask, mix 1 tablespoon of green clay with enough water to form a paste, adding a few drops of lavender essential oil for its calming effects. Apply the mask to your face, avoiding the eye area, and leave it on for 10-15 minutes before rinsing with warm water. This mask can help remove impurities, absorb excess oil, and improve skin texture with regular use. Green clay is particularly beneficial for oily and combination skin types.

By integrating these natural ingredients into your facial care routine, you can harness the power of plants to nourish, protect, and revitalize your skin. Each ingredient offers unique benefits, allowing you to customize your skincare regimen to address specific concerns and preferences. Whether you're looking to soothe irritation, hydrate dry skin, or combat acne, nature provides a wealth of solutions that can be tailored to meet your needs.

Herbal Face Masks and Scrubs

For a revitalizing **Honey and Papaya Face Mask**, begin by mashing half a ripe papaya until it forms a smooth paste. Papaya contains the enzyme papain, which exfoliates dead skin cells and aids in rejuvenating the skin's surface. Combine this with 1 tablespoon of raw honey, known for its antibacterial and moisturizing properties. Mix well. Apply the mask to your face, avoiding the eye area, and leave it on for 20 minutes. Rinse with lukewarm water. This mask is particularly beneficial for those looking to brighten and hydrate their skin, making it appear more youthful and radiant.

For an **Oatmeal and Green Tea Scrub**, start by grinding 2 tablespoons of oatmeal in a blender until it reaches a fine consistency. Oatmeal is gentle on the skin and offers soothing properties, making it ideal for sensitive skin types. Brew a strong cup of green tea and allow it to cool; green tea is rich in antioxidants that protect the skin from environmental stressors. Mix the ground oatmeal with 1 tablespoon of cooled green tea and 1 teaspoon of honey, creating a paste. If the mixture is too thick, add a little more green tea until you achieve the desired consistency. Gently massage the scrub onto your face in circular motions, then rinse with cool water. This scrub not only exfoliates but also nourishes the skin, leaving it soft and refreshed.

For those with oily or acne-prone skin, a **Clay and Apple Cider Vinegar (ACV) Mask** can be particularly effective. Mix 2 tablespoons of bentonite clay with equal parts of apple cider vinegar. ACV helps to balance the skin's pH and remove excess oil, while bentonite clay draws out impurities from the pores. Apply the mask to clean skin and leave it on for 10-15 minutes, or until it dries. Rinse with warm water. This mask can help to reduce the appearance of pores and control oil production with regular use.

A **Coffee and Coconut Oil Scrub** is perfect for stimulating circulation and smoothing the skin. Combine 2 tablespoons of finely ground coffee with 1 tablespoon of coconut oil. Coffee is a natural exfoliant and can help to tighten the skin, while coconut oil moisturizes and softens. Massage the scrub onto your face and neck in gentle, circular motions, then rinse with warm water. This scrub not only exfoliates but also leaves the skin feeling smooth and invigorated.

For a soothing and anti-inflammatory effect, try a **Cucumber and Aloe Vera Mask**. Blend half a cucumber with 2 tablespoons of aloe vera gel until smooth. Cucumber is known for its hydrating and calming properties, making it ideal for soothing irritated or sunburned skin. Aloe vera gel provides a cooling effect while also moisturizing the skin. Apply the mask to your face and leave it on for 15-20 minutes before rinsing with cool water. This mask is especially refreshing during the warmer months or after sun exposure.

Each of these herbal face masks and scrubs can be made with ingredients found in your kitchen or garden, offering a natural and cost-effective way to care for your skin. By selecting the right combination of ingredients for your skin type and concerns, you can create a personalized skincare routine that harnesses the power of nature to achieve a healthy, glowing complexion. Remember to perform a patch test on a small area of skin before applying any new product to your entire face, especially if you have sensitive skin or allergies.

Anti-Aging Herbal Treatments

Ginkgo Biloba stands out for its profound anti-aging benefits, particularly in enhancing skin elasticity and reducing the visibility of fine lines and wrinkles. To leverage Ginkgo Biloba's properties, prepare a skin toner by steeping 1 tablespoon of dried Ginkgo Biloba leaves in one cup of boiling water for 15 minutes. Strain the mixture and allow it to cool. Once cooled, apply the toner to your face with a clean cotton ball after cleansing. The antioxidant-rich compounds in Ginkgo Biloba, such as flavonoids and terpenoids, help combat oxidative stress, a key factor in skin aging. For optimal results, incorporate this toner into your evening skincare routine, allowing the skin to rejuvenate overnight.

Bilberry extract, another potent ingredient, offers significant benefits for aging skin by promoting collagen production and enhancing skin hydration. Create a bilberry serum by mixing 5 drops of bilberry extract with 1 ounce of hyaluronic acid serum. This combination provides a powerful defense against skin aging, delivering hydration and improving skin firmness. Apply this serum nightly to clean skin, gently patting it in to facilitate absorption. Bilberry's high concentration of anthocyanins, powerful antioxidants, aids in protecting the skin from environmental aggressors and reducing the appearance of age spots.

Gotu Kola, revered for its wound-healing and collagen-boosting properties, can be used to make an anti-aging face cream. Begin by infusing 1/4 cup of dried Gotu Kola leaves in 1/2 cup of coconut oil at low heat for 2 hours. Strain the oil and allow it to cool. In a separate container, gently heat 1/4 cup of shea butter until it melts, then combine it with the Gotu Kola-infused coconut oil. As the mixture cools, whisk in 10 drops of vitamin E oil, which acts as a natural preservative and adds additional antioxidant benefits. Store the cream in a clean, airtight container and apply it to your face and neck each night. Gotu Kola enhances skin's elasticity and firmness by stimulating collagen production, making it a valuable ingredient in combating the signs of aging.

For those targeting dark spots and uneven skin tone, licorice root extract serves as an effective natural remedy. To incorporate licorice root into your skincare regimen, prepare a brightening face mask by mixing

1 teaspoon of licorice root powder with 2 teaspoons of raw honey and a few drops of lemon juice. Apply the mask to clean skin, leaving it on for 20 minutes before rinsing with lukewarm water. The glabridin component of licorice root inhibits melanin production, helping to fade hyperpigmentation and even out skin tone. Utilize this mask twice a week for best results.

Lastly, harness the power of hibiscus, often referred to as the 'Botox plant', for its firming and lifting effects. Create a hibiscus facial mist by steeping 1 tablespoon of dried hibiscus petals in one cup of boiling water for 20 minutes. Strain the liquid and pour it into a spray bottle, adding a few drops of rosehip seed oil for an extra boost of hydration and vitamin C. Use this mist throughout the day to refresh your skin and provide a firming effect. The natural alpha-hydroxy acids (AHAs) in hibiscus help to exfoliate, promote cell renewal, and improve skin elasticity, making it an excellent addition to an anti-aging skincare routine.

By incorporating these herbal treatments into your skincare regimen, you can address various signs of aging through natural, effective means. Each herb offers unique benefits, allowing you to tailor your approach to meet your specific skin concerns. Regular use of these herbal preparations, combined with a healthy lifestyle, can significantly improve the health and appearance of your skin, revealing a more youthful, radiant complexion.

Herbal Hair Care

For a nourishing **Rosemary and Nettle Hair Rinse**, start by boiling 2 cups of water. Add 1 tablespoon of dried rosemary leaves and 1 tablespoon of dried nettle leaves to the boiling water. Rosemary stimulates the scalp and promotes hair growth, while nettle is rich in minerals that nourish the hair follicles. Reduce the heat and let the mixture simmer for 20 minutes. After simmering, remove from heat and let it cool to room temperature. Strain the mixture to remove the leaves. After shampooing, pour the rosemary and nettle rinse through your hair as a final rinse. Do not rinse out with water; allow your hair to air dry to absorb all the benefits. This rinse can be used once or twice a week to promote healthy hair growth and add shine.

To combat dry scalp and dandruff, prepare a **Coconut Oil and Tea Tree Scalp Treatment**. Begin by melting 2 tablespoons of coconut oil in a small saucepan over low heat. Coconut oil is deeply moisturizing and has antifungal properties that can help to combat dandruff. Once melted, remove from heat and stir in 5 drops of tea tree essential oil. Tea tree oil is known for its antibacterial and antifungal qualities, making it effective in treating dry scalp conditions. Allow the mixture to cool slightly, then massage it into your scalp. Leave the treatment on for at least 30 minutes, or overnight for more intense hydration. Wash your hair with a gentle shampoo to remove the oil. This treatment can be applied once a week to maintain a healthy scalp.

For a simple **Avocado and Honey Hair Mask**, mash one ripe avocado in a bowl. Avocado is rich in vitamins and minerals that are essential for healthy hair, including vitamins E and B. Add 1 tablespoon of honey to the mashed avocado. Honey is a natural humectant that attracts moisture, helping to hydrate dry hair. Mix the ingredients until you achieve a smooth paste. Apply the mask to damp hair, making sure to cover from roots to ends. Cover your hair with a shower cap and let the mask sit for 30 minutes. Rinse thoroughly with warm water and shampoo as usual. This mask can be used every two weeks to deeply moisturize the hair and enhance its natural shine.

To strengthen hair and prevent breakage, try a **Horsetail and Lavender Strengthening Spray**. Boil 2 cups of water and add 1 tablespoon of dried horsetail and 1 tablespoon of dried lavender. Horsetail is a source of silica, which is known to strengthen hair and improve its texture. Lavender adds a soothing scent and has properties that can promote hair growth. Let the mixture steep for 1 hour, then strain and pour the liquid into a spray bottle. Spray onto damp hair focusing on the ends, and comb through. Do not rinse out. The strengthening spray can be used after each wash to protect hair from breakage and maintain its health.

For increased hair volume, a **Peppermint and Green Tea Volumizing Rinse** can be very effective. Brew a strong cup of green tea and add 5 drops of peppermint essential oil to it once cooled. Green tea is rich in antioxidants that can stimulate hair follicles and promote growth, while peppermint oil invigorates the scalp, encouraging blood flow and resulting in fuller-looking hair. After shampooing, pour the rinse over your scalp and hair, massaging gently. Leave it on for 5 minutes, then rinse with cool water. This rinse can be used once a week to enhance volume and add a refreshing scent to your hair care routine.

By incorporating these herbal hair care treatments into your regimen, you can harness the power of natural ingredients to address a variety of hair concerns. From promoting growth and adding shine to treating scalp conditions and preventing breakage, these remedies offer a holistic approach to maintaining healthy, vibrant hair.

Natural Shampoos and Conditioners

Transitioning to natural shampoos and conditioners can be a significant step towards embracing a holistic approach to hair care. Unlike commercial products that often contain harsh chemicals and synthetic fragrances, natural alternatives nourish the scalp and hair using the therapeutic properties of herbs, essential oils, and other organic ingredients. This section delves into creating your own natural shampoos and conditioners, focusing on ingredients that promote hair health, cleanliness, and manageability.

For a basic natural shampoo, the foundation typically consists of a gentle, natural soap base, such as castile soap, which is derived from olive oil and known for its mild cleansing properties. To this base, you can add a variety of herbal infusions and essential oils tailored to your hair type and needs. For instance, a shampoo designed for oily hair might include rosemary and peppermint essential oils, both of which have astringent properties that help regulate oil production on the scalp. To prepare this shampoo, start by mixing 1/2 cup of liquid castile soap with 1/4 cup of distilled water. Then, add 2 tablespoons of a rosemary and peppermint herbal infusion, which you can make by steeping the dried herbs in boiling water for 30 minutes. Finally, incorporate 10 drops each of rosemary and peppermint essential oils into the mixture. This shampoo not only cleanses the hair but also stimulates the scalp, promoting healthy hair growth.

For dry or damaged hair, a moisturizing conditioner can be made by combining natural oils and butters that deeply hydrate and repair the hair shaft. A simple yet effective conditioner can be created using coconut oil, shea butter, and aloe vera gel. Begin by melting 2 tablespoons of coconut oil and 1 tablespoon of shea butter in a double boiler over low heat. Once melted, remove from heat and whisk in 1/4 cup of aloe vera gel, known for its soothing and moisturizing properties. To enhance the conditioner's benefits, add 5 drops of lavender essential oil, which not only adds a calming fragrance but also helps to soothe the scalp. Apply this conditioner to clean, damp hair, focusing on the ends where damage is most likely to occur. Leave it on for 5 minutes before rinsing thoroughly with warm water.

For those seeking to address specific scalp conditions such as dandruff, a targeted shampoo can be formulated using tea tree essential oil, renowned for its antifungal and antibacterial properties. Combine 1/2 cup of liquid castile soap with 1/4 cup of distilled water and 1 tablespoon of apple cider vinegar, which helps to balance the scalp's pH. Then, add 15 drops of tea tree essential oil. This shampoo can be used two to three times a week to help control dandruff and soothe scalp irritation.

Creating natural shampoos and conditioners allows for customization based on individual hair needs and preferences. It's important to note that natural hair care products may not produce the same lather as commercial ones but are just as effective at cleansing and conditioning the hair. Additionally, transitioning to natural hair care products may involve an adjustment period for the scalp and hair to rebalance its natural oil production.

When selecting ingredients for your natural shampoos and conditioners, always opt for high-quality, organic options to ensure the purity and efficacy of your hair care products. Essential oils should be therapeutic grade, and herbal infusions should be made from dried herbs that have not been treated with pesticides or chemicals. By taking the time to craft your own hair care products, you're not only taking a step towards healthier hair but also contributing to a more sustainable and environmentally friendly beauty regimen.

Herbal Rinses for Hair Health

For those seeking to enhance the luster and health of their hair through natural means, incorporating a Chamomile and Lemon Rinse can be remarkably effective, especially for lightening hair or adding highlights over time. To prepare this rinse, begin by boiling 2 cups of water. Add 1 tablespoon of dried chamomile flowers, known for their gentle lightening properties, and the juice of one lemon, which acts as a natural bleaching agent. Allow the mixture to simmer for 30 minutes, enabling the chamomile and lemon to infuse the water. After simmering, let the concoction cool, then strain to remove the chamomile flowers. Use this rinse after shampooing, pouring it evenly over your hair and scalp. Leave it in your hair without rinsing it out with water; the acidic nature of lemon juice can help close the hair cuticles, resulting in smoother, shinier hair. This rinse is particularly beneficial during the summer months when combined with sun exposure to naturally enhance highlights.

For individuals with darker hair or those looking to darken their hair naturally, a Sage and Rosemary Hair Rinse offers a traditional remedy to gradually deepen hair color and cover grays. Boil 2 cups of water and add 1 tablespoon each of dried sage and rosemary. Both herbs are revered for their ability to naturally darken hair over time and improve scalp health. Let the mixture simmer for 20-30 minutes, allowing the herbs to release their color and beneficial properties. After cooling and straining, apply the rinse to your hair post-shampooing. It's advisable to let your hair air dry to fully absorb the rinse. With regular use, you may notice a subtle deepening of your hair color and a vibrant, healthy sheen.

For scalp health, particularly to alleviate itchiness and dryness, a Calendula and Aloe Vera Scalp Rinse can offer soothing relief. Start by preparing an infusion of calendula by boiling 2 cups of water and steeping 1 tablespoon of dried calendula flowers for 30 minutes. Calendula is known for its anti-inflammatory and healing properties, making it ideal for sensitive or irritated scalps. After straining the calendula flowers, combine the infusion with 1/4 cup of pure aloe vera gel, which hydrates and soothes the scalp. Apply this mixture directly to the scalp after shampooing, gently massaging it in for several minutes before rinsing with cool water. This treatment can help to soothe scalp irritation, promote healing, and enhance overall scalp health with its hydrating and anti-inflammatory effects.

For hair that lacks strength and is prone to breakage, a Protein-Rich Gelatin Hair Mask can provide the necessary reinforcement. Dissolve 1 tablespoon of unflavored gelatin in 1 cup of warm water, stirring until fully dissolved to avoid lumps. Gelatin is rich in protein, which helps to strengthen the hair shaft and repair damage. Add 1 teaspoon of apple cider vinegar to balance the scalp's pH and 5 drops of lavender essential oil for its calming scent and scalp benefits. After shampooing, apply this mask to damp hair, leaving it on for 10 minutes before rinsing thoroughly with cool water. This treatment can be used once a month to fortify the hair, improve elasticity, and reduce breakage.

Incorporating these herbal rinses and treatments into your hair care routine can significantly improve the health, appearance, and vitality of your hair. By leveraging the natural properties of herbs and other natural ingredients, you can achieve desired hair qualities, from color enhancement to strength and shine, without relying on harsh chemicals. Regular use and patience are key, as natural remedies often require consistent application over time to manifest visible results.

Chapter 10: The Herbal Kitchen

Incorporating herbs into your cooking not only enhances flavor but also boosts the nutritional value of your meals. One of the simplest ways to start is by creating herbal oils and vinegars, which can be used in a myriad of recipes, from salad dressings to marinades. To make a basic herbal oil, choose a high-quality, organic carrier oil such as extra virgin olive oil or coconut oil for its health benefits and flavor profile. Select fresh herbs from your garden or local market—basil, rosemary, and thyme are excellent choices for their robust flavors and health properties.

Begin by gently bruising the herbs to release their essential oils, a crucial step to infuse the carrier oil with flavor and nutrients. You can do this by lightly crushing them with a mortar and pestle or rolling them with a rolling pin. Next, place the bruised herbs in a clean, dry jar and pour the carrier oil over them, ensuring the herbs are completely submerged to prevent mold growth. Seal the jar tightly and store it in a cool, dark place for 1-2 weeks, shaking it gently every few days to distribute the flavors. After the infusion period, strain the oil through a fine mesh sieve or cheesecloth to remove the herbs. The resulting herbal oil can be stored in a clean, airtight container in a cool, dark place for up to a month.

For herbal vinegars, apple cider vinegar is a popular choice due to its health benefits, including digestive support and blood sugar regulation. The process is similar to making herbal oils. Start with fresh herbs—dill, mint, and tarragon work wonderfully for their distinct flavors. Rinse the herbs and pat them dry to remove any moisture, which could spoil the vinegar. Place the herbs in a clean jar and cover them with apple cider vinegar. Seal the jar and store it in a cool, dark place, allowing it to infuse for 2-4 weeks. Remember to shake the jar occasionally to mix the herbs. Once infused to your liking, strain the vinegar to remove the herbs, and bottle the vinegar for use. It can be stored at room temperature and used within a year.

These infused oils and vinegars can serve as the base for dressings, marinades, or to add a flavorful touch to cooked dishes. The beauty of these infusions lies in their simplicity and the ability to customize them according to your taste preferences and the seasonal availability of herbs.

Expanding beyond oils and vinegars, herbal salts and sugars offer another dimension to your culinary palette, allowing you to incorporate the healing and aromatic properties of herbs into every aspect of your cooking and baking. To create an herbal salt, finely chop fresh herbs such as rosemary, lavender, or sage, and mix them with high-quality sea salt or Himalayan pink salt. The ratio of herbs to salt can vary depending on personal preference, but a good starting point is one part herb to three parts salt. Spread the mixture on a baking sheet and allow it to dry in a warm, well-ventilated area or in an oven set to the lowest possible temperature. Once dry, store the herbal salt in an airtight container. Use it to season dishes, as a finishing salt, or even as a rim for cocktail glasses to add an unexpected herbal note.

Herbal sugars can be created in a similar fashion, using either granulated sugar or a finer caster sugar for a more delicate texture. Lavender, rose petals, and mint are excellent choices for infusing sugar. The process mirrors that of making herbal salt, with the herb-to-sugar ratio adjusted to taste. Herbal sugars are perfect for baking, sweetening teas and coffees, or sprinkling over fresh fruit for a gourmet touch.

For those interested in exploring the medicinal benefits of herbs in their cooking, creating healing herbal broths is an excellent way to start. These broths can serve as a base for soups, stews, or as a comforting drink. Begin with a selection of herbs known for their health-supporting properties, such as nettle for its iron content, dandelion for detoxification, and ginger for its digestive aid. Combine these with vegetables like carrots, celery, and onions to create a nutrient-rich broth. Cover with water and simmer gently for several hours, allowing the flavors and properties of the herbs to infuse the liquid. Strain the broth and use immediately, or store in the refrigerator for up to a week. You can also freeze the broth in ice cube trays for easy use in future recipes.

Lastly, the art of making homemade herbal wines and cordials is a delightful way to preserve the flavors and benefits of herbs. Dandelion wine, elderflower cordial, and rose petal wine are just a few examples of the myriad possibilities. These beverages require more time and patience but offer a unique way to enjoy the bounty of your herbal garden. Start with fresh or dried herbs, sugar, and a base such as water for cordials or a grape or apple juice for wines. The fermentation process will vary depending on the recipe, but the result is a homemade creation that captures the essence of the herbs in a form that can be enjoyed by adults in moderation.

Incorporating herbs into your kitchen practices not only enhances the flavor of your food but also imbues your meals with the natural health benefits of these powerful plants. Whether through simple infusions, elaborate broths, or the creation of herbal condiments, the possibilities are endless. By harnessing the flavors and medicinal properties of herbs, you can transform your kitchen into a place of healing, comfort, and culinary exploration.

Cooking with Herbs

Herbal spices and seasonings are a cornerstone of creating flavorful and healthful dishes in the herbal kitchen. To craft your own herbal seasonings, start by selecting fresh herbs that complement the dishes you frequently cook. Popular choices include basil, oregano, thyme, rosemary, and sage. These herbs not only impart unique flavors but also offer various health benefits, from anti-inflammatory properties to aiding digestion.

Drying Herbs

To preserve the potency of your herbs, drying them is a necessary step. Begin by washing the herbs gently to remove any dirt or debris. Pat them dry with a clean towel or use a salad spinner to remove excess moisture. Next, tie the stems of the herbs together and hang them upside down in a warm, dry area away from direct sunlight. This could be in an attic, a pantry, or even a kitchen corner that does not receive much sunlight. The drying process can take anywhere from a week to several weeks, depending on the humidity and air circulation in your drying area. Once the herbs are completely dry, their leaves should crumble easily between your fingers.

Creating Herbal Seasoning Blends

After drying, the next step is to create your seasoning blends. Using a mortar and pestle or a spice grinder, crush the dried herbs into a fine powder. This method allows you to control the texture of the seasoning, whether you prefer it finely ground or slightly coarse. For a simple Italian seasoning blend, combine equal parts of dried basil, oregano, rosemary, and thyme. Store your herbal seasoning in an airtight container, away from heat and light, to maintain its freshness and potency.

Herbal Salts

To make herbal salts, mix one part of your ground, dried herbs with three parts of coarse sea salt or Himalayan pink salt. This not only flavors the salt but also incorporates the health benefits of the herbs into your cooking. Herbal salts are perfect for seasoning meats, vegetables, or for finishing dishes right before serving.

Herbal Sugars

For desserts or sweetening beverages, herbal sugars are an excellent addition to your pantry. Combine finely ground dried herbs such as lavender, rose petals, or mint with granulated sugar. The ratio of herbs to sugar can be adjusted according to taste, but a starting point is one part herb to four parts sugar. Use a food processor to blend the herbs and sugar together until well mixed. Store in an airtight container and use to sweeten teas, coffees, or sprinkle over baked goods for a subtle herbal flavor.

Using Fresh Herbs

While dried herbs are great for seasoning blends and long-term storage, fresh herbs offer a burst of flavor that can elevate any dish. When using fresh herbs, add them towards the end of the cooking process to preserve their flavor and nutritional value. For instance, fresh basil can be torn and sprinkled over a finished pasta dish, or fresh cilantro can be added to a taco filling just before serving.

Infusing Oils with Herbs

Another method to incorporate herbs into your cooking is by infusing oils. Choose a high-quality oil such as extra virgin olive oil, and add fresh or dried herbs of your choice. Warm the oil gently with the herbs over low heat for 5-10 minutes, then allow it to cool. Strain the oil to remove the herbs, and store the infused oil in a clean, airtight bottle. Use these infused oils as a base for salad dressings, marinades, or as a simple dip for fresh bread.

Incorporating herbs into your cooking not only enhances the taste of your food but also boosts its nutritional profile. By creating your own herbal seasonings, salts, and sugars, you can add a personal touch to your dishes while reaping the health benefits that these natural ingredients offer. Whether you're using fresh or dried herbs, the key is to experiment with different combinations and find what works best for your palate and cooking style.

Infusing Oils and Vinegars

When delving into the process of infusing oils and vinegars, the precision in selecting the right ingredients and following a meticulous method cannot be overstated. The quality of the base oil or vinegar directly influences the final product's flavor, aroma, and health benefits. For oils, opting for a high-quality, organic carrier oil such as extra virgin olive oil, coconut oil, or almond oil is essential. These oils not only provide a robust foundation for the infusion but also contribute their own health benefits, ranging from heart-healthy fats in olive oil to the moisturizing properties of coconut oil. Similarly, when choosing vinegar as a base, apple cider vinegar stands out for its health-promoting properties, including enhancing digestion and supporting a healthy immune system, though white wine vinegar and rice vinegar also serve as excellent canvases for infusion due to their subtle, nuanced flavors.

The selection of herbs is equally crucial, with freshness and quality taking precedence. The herbs must be thoroughly washed and completely dried to remove any moisture, as the presence of water can lead to spoilage or mold growth during the infusion process. For oils, robust, hardy herbs such as rosemary, thyme, and oregano are ideal, as their flavors infuse well into the oil without becoming overpowering. For vinegars, more delicate herbs like basil, dill, and mint can be used, as the acidic nature of vinegar can better preserve their fresh, vibrant flavors.

The technique for infusing oils involves gently bruising the selected herbs to begin releasing their essential oils, a critical step for transferring the herbs' essence into the carrier oil. This can be achieved by using a mortar and pestle or by simply pressing the herbs with the back of a spoon. The bruised herbs are then submerged in the carrier oil in a clean, dry jar, ensuring that the herbs are fully covered to prevent any exposure to air, which could lead to oxidation and spoilage. The jar should be sealed tightly and stored in a cool, dark place for a period of 1 to 2 weeks, depending on the desired strength of the infusion. It's important to shake the jar gently every few days to ensure the herbs' flavors are evenly distributed throughout the oil.

For vinegar infusions, the process is similar, with the clean, dry herbs placed in a jar and covered with vinegar. The jar is then sealed and stored in a cool, dark place. However, the infusion time for vinegar can be shorter, ranging from 2 to 4 weeks, as the acidic environment of the vinegar extracts the flavors and medicinal properties of the herbs more efficiently. Regular shaking of the jar is also recommended to facilitate even flavor distribution.

After the infusion period, the next critical step is straining the oil or vinegar to remove the herbs. This should be done using a fine mesh sieve or cheesecloth to ensure that all plant material is removed, leaving behind a clear, infused liquid. The strained oil or vinegar should then be transferred to a clean, airtight container for storage. Infused oils should be stored in a cool, dark place and used within a month to maintain freshness and prevent rancidity. Infused vinegars can be stored at room temperature and have a longer shelf life, typically up to a year, due to vinegar's natural preservative properties.

The resulting infused oils and vinegars are not only a testament to the art of infusion but also a versatile addition to any culinary repertoire. They can be used to elevate the flavor of salads, marinades, and cooked dishes, adding a layer of complexity and depth with the subtle nuances of the infused herbs. Moreover, these infusions embody the essence of the herbs' medicinal properties, offering a holistic approach to cooking that aligns with the principles of natural wellness and health self-sufficiency.

In crafting these infusions, attention to detail, patience, and a willingness to experiment with different herb combinations are key. Each batch of infused oil or vinegar is a unique creation, reflecting the individual tastes and preferences of the creator and the seasonal availability of herbs. Through this process, one not only enhances their culinary creations but also deepens their connection to the natural world and the ancient traditions of herbal medicine.

Herbal Spices and Seasonings

Incorporating herbal spices and seasonings into your culinary practices not only enriches the flavor palette of your dishes but also imbues them with health-enhancing properties, seamlessly blending the art of cooking with the science of wellness. The process of selecting and combining herbs for your seasoning blends requires a thoughtful approach, taking into consideration the flavor profiles of each herb and how they complement each other as well as the dishes they will season.

When creating herbal seasoning blends, consider the culinary traditions and flavor profiles you enjoy. For instance, a blend inspired by Mediterranean cuisine might focus on herbs such as oregano, thyme, and marjoram, known for their robust flavors and compatibility with olive oil-based dishes. On the other hand, a blend leaning towards French cuisine could emphasize herbs like tarragon, chervil, and lavender, offering a more delicate and nuanced flavor suitable for sauces and poultry dishes.

The technique of blending herbs involves more than simply mixing different herbs together. It requires an understanding of each herb's flavor intensity and how it evolves during the cooking process. Hardy herbs like rosemary and sage have a strong presence and can withstand long cooking times, making them ideal for inclusion in blends intended for roasting or grilling. Conversely, delicate herbs such as cilantro and parsley are best added towards the end of cooking or used in fresh applications to preserve their vibrant color and flavor.

To create a balanced herbal blend, start with a base of neutral-flavored herbs like parsley or thyme, then add smaller quantities of more potent herbs for depth and complexity. This method ensures that no single flavor overpowers the others, allowing for a harmonious blend that enhances rather than competes with the natural flavors of the food.

For those interested in exploring the therapeutic aspects of culinary herbs, incorporating adaptogenic herbs into seasoning blends offers a way to enhance the body's resilience to stress. Herbs such as holy basil (tulsi) and ashwagandha can be finely ground and added in small amounts to everyday seasoning blends, providing a subtle, health-supportive boost to meals.

Storage and preservation of herbal spices and seasonings are critical to maintaining their potency and flavor. After blending, store your herbal seasonings in airtight containers, labeled with the date of creation. Keep them in a cool, dark cupboard to protect against light and heat, which can degrade the essential oils responsible for the herbs' flavors and medicinal properties. Properly stored, dry herbal blends can retain their quality for up to a year, though it's best to use them within six months for maximum freshness.

In utilizing these herbal spices and seasonings, start with small amounts to gauge their impact on your dishes, keeping in mind that the goal is to complement and enhance the natural flavors of your ingredients. Over time, you may find yourself adjusting the proportions of herbs in your blends to suit your taste preferences and health goals, embracing the dynamic nature of cooking with herbs.

By integrating herbal spices and seasonings into your culinary repertoire, you not only elevate the taste and nutritional profile of your meals but also deepen your connection to the natural world. This practice invites a mindful approach to cooking and eating, where each meal becomes an opportunity to nourish and heal the body, aligning with the principles of holistic wellness and self-sufficiency.

Herbal Beverages and Elixirs

Herbal beverages and elixirs offer a delightful and healthful addition to your daily routine, providing both hydration and therapeutic benefits. To create these nourishing drinks, start by selecting high-quality, organic herbs known for their medicinal properties. For a calming tea, chamomile and lavender are excellent choices, while ginger and turmeric are ideal for an anti-inflammatory tonic. The process of making herbal teas involves steeping the chosen herbs in boiling water for a specified period, usually between 5 to 15 minutes, depending on the desired strength and the herb's characteristics. For a more potent elixir, consider decoction, a method where the herbs are simmered in water over low heat for a longer duration, typically 20 minutes to several hours, effectively extracting the deeper essences and beneficial compounds of tougher roots, barks, and berries.

Cold Infusions are another method, particularly suited for delicate herbs or when seeking a refreshing beverage. Simply place the herbs in a jar filled with cold water and let them infuse overnight in the refrigerator. This slow extraction process preserves the subtle flavors and therapeutic qualities of the herbs without the bitterness that heat can sometimes introduce.

Herbal Syrups provide a sweet, concentrated form of herbal benefits and can be added to hot water, teas, or carbonated water for a quick herbal soda. To make a simple syrup, combine equal parts water and sugar in a saucepan, bring to a simmer, and then add your chosen herbs. Let the mixture simmer for 30 minutes, then strain and bottle the syrup. For added preservation, a splash of brandy or vodka can extend the shelf life.

When crafting **Herbal Elixirs**, blending herbs with alcohol can extract both water-soluble and alcohol-soluble compounds, making them more potent than teas or decoctions. Start with a clean jar and fill it one-third to one-half with dried herbs. Cover the herbs with a neutral spirit such as vodka or brandy, ensuring the herbs are completely submerged. Seal the jar and store it in a cool, dark place, shaking it daily for 4 to 6 weeks. After this period, strain the liquid, and your elixir is ready to be used. These elixirs can be taken in small doses, typically a teaspoon at a time, either directly or diluted in water.

For a **Herbal Kombucha**, begin with a base of green or black tea, sweetened with sugar, and then introduce a SCOBY (Symbiotic Culture Of Bacteria and Yeast). After the initial fermentation, add your chosen herbs during the second fermentation process to infuse the kombucha with their flavors and benefits. Popular choices include ginger for digestion, hibiscus for its antioxidant properties, and lavender for relaxation. Monitor the taste and carbonation level daily until it reaches your desired potency, usually within 3 to 7 days, then refrigerate to stop fermentation.

Golden Milk, a traditional Ayurvedic drink, involves simmering turmeric with milk (dairy or plant-based) and a touch of black pepper to enhance absorption. Sweeten with honey or maple syrup and add a pinch of cinnamon or cardamom for extra flavor and warmth. This beverage is particularly beneficial for its anti-inflammatory and antioxidant properties.

In creating these herbal beverages and elixirs, always use filtered water to ensure the cleanest possible base free from chlorine and other chemicals that could interfere with the flavors and medicinal qualities of the herbs. Additionally, when working with fresh herbs, ensure they are thoroughly washed and free from pesticides and contaminants. The choice of sweeteners can vary according to taste and dietary preferences, with natural options like honey, maple syrup, or stevia being healthier alternatives to refined sugar.

By incorporating these herbal beverages and elixirs into your daily routine, you can enjoy the myriad flavors and health benefits that herbs offer. Whether seeking relaxation, immune support, or digestive aid, there is a herbal drink to meet your needs. Experiment with different herbs and combinations to discover your personal favorites and to tailor your concoctions to specific health goals.

Homemade Herbal Wines and Cordials

Creating homemade herbal wines and cordials is an enriching process that combines the art of fermentation with the healing properties of herbs, offering a unique way to enjoy the benefits of herbal remedies. The process begins with selecting high-quality, organic herbs that complement the flavor profile of the base wine or spirit and enhance its medicinal value. For herbal wines, consider herbs like elderflower, dandelion, or rose petals for their floral notes and health benefits. Elderflower, for instance, is known for its immune-boosting properties, while dandelion can support liver health. For cordials, robust herbs such as ginger, turmeric, or hibiscus can be used to create a potent and flavorful tonic that can aid digestion, reduce inflammation, or provide antioxidant benefits.

The first step in making herbal wine is to prepare a base wine, which can be a simple country wine made from fruits such as grapes, apples, or berries. The fruit is fermented with water, sugar, and yeast until it reaches the desired alcohol content and flavor profile. Once the base wine is ready, the selected herbs are added. The herbs can be infused directly into the wine by adding them to the fermenting vessel during the secondary fermentation process. This allows the alcohol to extract the flavors and medicinal properties of the herbs over time. The quantity of herbs used should be carefully measured to avoid overpowering the wine; typically, a ratio of one part herb to ten parts wine by volume is a good starting point.

For herbal cordials, the process involves creating a strong infusion or decoction of the chosen herbs in water, which is then mixed with a spirit such as vodka, brandy, or rum. The spirit acts as a preservative, extending the shelf life of the cordial and extracting a broader range of medicinal compounds from the herbs. The herb-to-water ratio is crucial here, with a general guideline being one part herb to four parts water for infusions, or one part herb to two parts water for decoctions. After the herbs have been steeped and the liquid strained, it is mixed with the spirit and sweetened with honey, sugar, or another natural sweetener to taste. The sweetness not only improves the flavor but also helps to meld the herbal and alcoholic components into a harmonious blend.

The aging process is vital for both herbal wines and cordials, allowing the flavors to meld and mature. Herbal wines can benefit from aging for several months to a year, while cordials may be ready to consume after a few weeks of aging, though longer aging can enhance their complexity and depth of flavor. During aging, the containers should be stored in a cool, dark place to prevent oxidation and preserve the delicate herbal notes.

Bottling is the final step, requiring sterilized bottles and airtight seals to ensure the longevity and safety of the herbal wine or cordial. It's important to label each bottle with the type of herb used, the date of bottling, and any other relevant information, such as the intended use or dosage recommendations. This meticulous record-keeping not only adds a professional touch but also helps in tracking the effectiveness and preferences for future batches.

When enjoyed in moderation, homemade herbal wines and cordials can serve as a delightful addition to a holistic wellness regimen, offering both pleasure and health benefits. The process of creating these beverages encourages a deeper connection with the natural world, a creative exploration of flavors, and a commitment to health that is both rewarding and enjoyable. Whether sipping a glass of dandelion wine on a warm summer evening or enjoying a ginger-infused cordial as a winter tonic, the art of making homemade herbal wines and cordials is a fulfilling way to integrate the healing power of herbs into everyday life.

Healing Herbal Broths

Healing herbal broths serve as a foundational element in the holistic family apothecary, offering a versatile and nourishing way to incorporate medicinal herbs into your daily diet. These broths can be tailored to address specific health concerns or to provide general wellness support. The process begins with selecting **high-quality, organic herbs** and combining them with a variety of vegetables to create a rich, flavorful base.

To start, choose a **large stainless-steel or ceramic pot** to ensure even heat distribution and prevent any interaction with the herbs. Begin by gently sautéing a mirepoix of onions, carrots, and celery in a small amount of **extra virgin olive oil**. This not only lays the groundwork for flavor but also starts the release of beneficial nutrients.

For the herbal component, consider herbs such as **reishi mushrooms** for immune support, **nettle leaves** for their rich mineral content, or **dandelion root** for liver detoxification. It's important to use a **muslin bag or a large tea infuser** to contain the herbs, making them easy to remove after cooking.
Add cold, filtered water to the pot, ensuring the water covers the vegetables and herbs by at least 2 inches. This ratio allows for the maximum extraction of nutrients and flavors. Bring the broth to a gentle simmer, never allowing it to reach a rolling boil, as high heat can destroy some of the delicate compounds in the herbs.
Simmer the broth for a minimum of **2 hours**, though longer cooking times of up to 4 hours may be beneficial for extracting deeper flavors and more potent medicinal properties. If adding tougher roots or barks, such as **astragalus root** for additional immune support, these can be added at the beginning of the cooking process as they withstand longer cooking times well.
Throughout the simmering process, periodically check the water level, adding more as needed to maintain the original volume. This ensures that the broth remains concentrated and full of flavor.
Once the broth has finished cooking, remove it from the heat and allow it to cool slightly. Carefully strain the broth through a fine-mesh sieve or cheesecloth to remove all solid materials, pressing gently on the vegetables and herbs to extract their full essence.
For additional flavor and health benefits, consider stirring in a teaspoon of **organic miso paste** after the broth has cooled slightly. Miso, being a fermented product, adds beneficial probiotics to the broth, but it should not be boiled to preserve its live cultures.

The final broth can be seasoned to taste with **Himalayan pink salt** or **sea salt** and **black pepper**, but keep the seasoning light to allow the natural flavors of the herbs and vegetables to shine through.

Herbal broths can be consumed on their own or used as a base for soups, stews, and grains, making them a versatile addition to the holistic kitchen. For storage, allow the broth to cool completely before transferring it to **glass jars or BPA-free containers**. It can be stored in the refrigerator for up to 5 days or frozen for up to 3 months for longer preservation.

By integrating healing herbal broths into your family's diet, you are taking a proactive step towards nurturing health and wellness through the power of nature's pharmacy. Each sip provides a comforting and healing embrace, supporting the body's natural healing processes and offering a daily dose of preventative care.

Chapter 11: Gardening for Your Apothecary

Creating a medicinal garden for your home apothecary is a rewarding endeavor that not only beautifies your space but also serves as a vital resource for natural health and wellness. The process begins with planning and selecting the right location in your garden. A successful medicinal garden requires careful consideration of sunlight, soil quality, and water access. Most medicinal herbs thrive in a location that receives at least six hours of direct sunlight daily. The ideal soil for a medicinal garden is well-draining and rich in organic matter. If your garden soil is heavy clay or sandy, it can be improved by incorporating compost or aged manure to enhance its structure and fertility.

Water access is crucial for establishing young plants and sustaining them during dry periods. While many herbs are drought-tolerant once established, consistent moisture is important in the early stages of growth. Consider installing a drip irrigation system or soaker hoses to provide a steady, efficient water supply directly to the plant roots, minimizing waste and reducing the risk of leaf diseases that can occur with overhead watering.

When selecting herbs for your garden, consider both your family's health needs and the growing conditions of your area. Start with easy-to-grow herbs such as **chamomile**, **mint**, **lavender**, and **calendula**, which offer a wide range of medicinal benefits from calming teas to healing salves. Research the specific needs of each herb, as some may require special conditions, such as the cooler, shaded environment preferred by **lemon balm** or the dry, well-drained soil favored by **sage** and **thyme**.

Incorporating perennials like **echinacea** and **valerian** alongside annuals and biennials ensures a diverse, year-round supply of medicinal plants. Perennials provide the backbone of the medicinal garden, returning each year with minimal maintenance, while annuals and biennials can be rotated or changed each season to meet specific health interests or to try new remedies.

Designing your garden with companion planting in mind can enhance the health and yield of your medicinal plants. For example, planting **basil** near your **tomatoes** can improve their flavor and growth, while **marigolds** can deter pests from more vulnerable herbs. This approach not only maximizes the use of space but also promotes a balanced ecosystem in your garden, reducing the need for chemical pesticides and fertilizers.

Labeling each herb with its common and botanical name, along with its primary uses, can be a helpful reference as you harvest and utilize your plants. Creating a planting and harvesting calendar based on your specific climate and the growth cycles of your herbs will ensure that you make the most of your apothecary garden throughout the growing season. This calendar should include key dates for sowing seeds indoors, transplanting seedlings outside, and the optimal times for harvesting each herb to capture its maximum potency.

As you plan and plant your garden, consider the space each herb will need as it grows to maturity. Some herbs, like **mint**, are vigorous growers and can become invasive if not contained. Planting them in buried pots or designated areas can prevent them from overtaking your garden. On the other hand, delicate herbs such as **chamomile** may benefit from the support of neighboring plants or structures to protect them from strong winds or heavy rains.

In the next section, we will delve deeper into the specifics of soil preparation, pest management, and advanced techniques for maximizing the yield and potency of your medicinal herbs.

Soil preparation is a fundamental step in creating a thriving medicinal garden. Begin by testing your soil to determine its pH and nutrient levels. Most herbs prefer a slightly acidic to neutral pH, ranging from 6.0 to 7.0. If your soil is too acidic or alkaline, it can be amended with lime to raise the pH or sulfur to lower it. Incorporating organic matter such as compost not only improves soil structure and drainage but also provides essential nutrients to your plants. For raised beds or container gardens, a mix of one-third peat moss, one-third vermiculite or perlite, and one-third compost creates an ideal, well-draining growing medium for herbs.

Pest management in the medicinal garden should prioritize organic and sustainable practices to maintain the purity and efficacy of your herbs. Regular inspection of plants for signs of pests and disease is crucial for early intervention. Natural deterrents such as neem oil, diatomaceous earth, and insecticidal soaps can be effective against common pests while being safe for both the environment and your family. Encouraging beneficial insects like ladybugs, lacewings, and bees by planting a variety of flowers and herbs can help control pest populations naturally.

To maximize the yield and potency of your medicinal herbs, consider the timing of your harvest. Many herbs reach their peak medicinal value just before flowering when the concentration of essential oils is highest. Harvesting in the morning after the dew has evaporated but before the sun becomes too intense ensures that the herbs retain their aromatic oils and medicinal properties. Drying herbs properly is also critical for preserving their potency. Herbs can be air-dried in a warm, well-ventilated area away from direct sunlight or in a dehydrator set to a low temperature to maintain their therapeutic qualities.

Advanced techniques such as succession planting and crop rotation can further enhance the productivity of your medicinal garden. Succession planting involves staggering the planting of crops at regular intervals to ensure a continuous supply of herbs throughout the growing season. Crop rotation, on the other hand, involves changing the location of herbs each year to prevent soil depletion and reduce the build-up of pests and diseases. This practice not only supports the health of your garden but also encourages a diverse ecosystem.

In addition to these practices, creating microclimates within your garden can cater to the specific needs of certain herbs. For example, herbs that prefer a moist environment can be planted in lower areas of the garden where water collects, while those requiring drier conditions can be placed in raised beds or on slopes for better drainage. Utilizing mulches such as straw, bark, or leaf litter can help maintain soil moisture, regulate temperature, and suppress weed growth, benefiting your medicinal plants.

Remember, the key to a successful medicinal garden lies in understanding and catering to the unique needs of each herb. With careful planning, preparation, and maintenance, you can create a beautiful and productive space that provides a wealth of medicinal benefits for your family. By embracing these principles and practices, you'll not only cultivate a garden but also nurture your family's health and well-being through the power of nature's pharmacy.

Planning Your Medicinal Garden

To ensure your medicinal garden flourishes, focusing on **soil health** is paramount. Begin with a comprehensive soil test available from your local extension service to ascertain nutrient levels and pH balance. Most medicinal herbs thrive in a pH range of **6.0 to 7.0**. If your soil tests outside this range, adjust accordingly using lime to raise the pH or sulfur to lower it. This step is crucial because the correct pH ensures nutrient availability to your plants, directly impacting their medicinal qualities.

Incorporate generous amounts of **organic matter** into your garden beds. Well-composted organic matter not only improves soil structure and drainage but also adds essential nutrients. A healthy soil structure allows for better root growth and water retention, critical factors for the robust growth of herbs. For raised beds or containers, a mix of one-third peat moss, one-third vermiculite or perlite, and one-third compost provides an ideal environment for most herbs, ensuring good drainage and aeration.

Pest management requires a proactive and organic approach to preserve the integrity of your medicinal herbs. Start by selecting disease-resistant plant varieties and practice crop rotation to prevent soil-borne diseases. Employ physical barriers such as row covers to protect plants from pests. Introduce beneficial insects, like ladybugs and lacewings, by planting a diversity of flowers and herbs that attract them. For fungal issues, neem oil and baking soda sprays offer an organic solution without introducing harmful chemicals into your garden.

Watering practices play a significant role in the health of your medicinal garden. Overhead watering can spread diseases, so opt for drip irrigation or soaker hoses to deliver water directly to the base of the plants.

This method reduces water waste and minimizes the risk of leaf diseases. Water in the early morning to allow foliage to dry before evening, reducing the likelihood of fungal diseases.

Mulching is beneficial for maintaining soil moisture, regulating soil temperature, and suppressing weeds. Organic mulches, such as straw or shredded leaves, add nutrients to the soil as they decompose. Apply a 2 to 3-inch layer around your plants, keeping the mulch a few inches away from plant stems to prevent rot.

Harvesting your herbs at the right time is crucial for maximizing their medicinal properties. Most herbs are best harvested just before flowering when their essential oil content is highest. Harvest in the morning after the dew has evaporated but before the midday sun, which ensures the highest concentration of active constituents. Use sharp, clean scissors or pruners to make clean cuts, which helps the plants recover quickly.

Drying is a common method for preserving herbs, and doing it correctly is vital to maintain their medicinal qualities. Herbs can be air-dried in a warm, well-ventilated area away from direct sunlight. Alternatively, a dehydrator set to a low temperature can be used for more consistent results. Ensure herbs are completely dry before storing in airtight containers to prevent mold growth.

Labeling your plants and harvests with their common and botanical names, as well as harvest dates, ensures you use the correct plant part at the right time for remedies. This practice is especially important for beginners who are still familiarizing themselves with different herbs.

By implementing these detailed practices, you create a strong foundation for a productive and sustainable medicinal garden. Each step, from soil preparation to pest management and harvesting, contributes to the overall health and potency of your medicinal herbs, ensuring they can provide the maximum benefit for your family's health needs.

Selecting Herbs for Your Climate

Selecting the right herbs for your climate involves understanding the unique environmental conditions of your area, including temperature ranges, humidity levels, and the length of growing seasons. This knowledge enables you to choose herbs that will thrive in your garden, ensuring a bountiful and healthy apothecary. Begin by consulting the USDA Plant Hardiness Zone Map, which categorizes regions based on their average annual minimum winter temperature. This map serves as a fundamental guide for determining which plants are most likely to succeed in your locale.

For gardeners in cooler northern climates, zones 3 through 6, focus on hardy perennial herbs such as echinacea, which is renowned for its immune-boosting properties, and valerian, known for aiding sleep. These herbs can withstand cold winters and return year after year. Incorporating mulch around these plants will provide additional insulation against freezing temperatures, ensuring their roots are protected during the coldest months. It's also beneficial to select varieties that have been bred for cold tolerance and to consider using cold frames or hoop houses to extend the growing season.

In contrast, gardeners in warmer southern climates, zones 7 through 10, have a wider selection of herbs that can thrive due to the longer growing season and milder winters. Herbs such as lemon balm, sage, and thyme not only flourish in these conditions but can often be harvested year-round. However, these warmer regions may also experience intense heat and humidity, which can be challenging for some herbs. To mitigate these conditions, choose heat-tolerant varieties and employ strategies such as providing afternoon shade, using mulch to retain soil moisture, and ensuring adequate water to prevent stress from high temperatures.

For those in transitional zones, where temperatures can fluctuate widely, versatility in plant selection is key. Herbs like chamomile and mint are adaptable to a range of conditions, making them excellent choices for these areas. Mint, in particular, is vigorous and can adapt to various environments, but it's advisable to plant it in containers to control its spread. Additionally, employing a layered approach to planting, with taller plants providing shade for those that require cooler temperatures, can create microclimates within your garden, allowing a broader range of herbs to thrive.

Understanding your local soil type is another critical factor in selecting herbs for your climate. While most herbs prefer well-draining soil with a neutral pH, some, like lavender, require sandy, low-fertility soil to produce their best fragrance and medicinal qualities. If your soil does not naturally meet these conditions, amendments such as sand for drainage or organic matter to increase fertility can create a more suitable growing environment.

Watering practices must also be tailored to your climate. In arid regions, drip irrigation systems can deliver water directly to the root zone of plants, minimizing evaporation and ensuring that herbs receive the moisture they need without wasting water. In contrast, areas with abundant rainfall may require raised beds or well-draining soil amendments to prevent herbs from becoming waterlogged.

Finally, consider the ecological benefits of native herbs, which are naturally adapted to your climate and can provide habitat and food for local wildlife. Incorporating these plants into your garden supports biodiversity and can make your medicinal garden a haven for beneficial insects and birds. Native herbs often require less maintenance and are more resistant to pests and diseases, making them an excellent choice for the sustainable apothecary garden.

By carefully selecting herbs suited to your climate, employing strategies to mitigate extreme weather conditions, and adapting your gardening practices to the needs of your plants, you can cultivate a thriving medicinal garden that provides a wealth of health benefits for your family. This approach not only ensures the success of your apothecary garden but also fosters a deeper connection with the natural world and the cycles of the seasons.

Companion Planting and Permaculture Principles

Companion planting and permaculture principles are integral to creating a sustainable and productive medicinal garden. By understanding and implementing these strategies, you can enhance the health and yield of your herbs, reduce the need for chemical inputs, and create a garden that is in harmony with nature.

Companion Planting: This method involves planting different herbs and plants together to benefit each other. For example, **marigolds** emit a substance from their roots that deters nematodes, protecting neighboring plants like **tomatoes** and **basil**. Similarly, **chives** can improve the growth and flavor of **carrots** and **tomatoes** while deterring pests such as aphids. When planning your garden, consider the following companion planting combinations specifically beneficial for medicinal herbs:

- **Basil** with **chamomile** and **calendula**: Basil helps repel flies and mosquitoes, while chamomile improves its flavor and growth. Calendula attracts beneficial insects and can help protect basil from harmful pests.
- **Lavender** near **rosemary** and **sage**: These herbs share similar watering and sunlight needs, making them ideal companions. Lavender also attracts pollinators, which benefits the entire garden.
- **Mint** should be planted in containers to prevent it from becoming invasive. Place these containers near **roses** and **cabbages** to deter pests like aphids and cabbage moths.

When implementing companion planting, ensure that each plant's growth requirements, such as sunlight, water, and soil pH, are compatible. This approach not only maximizes space but also promotes a healthier, more diverse garden ecosystem.

Permaculture Principles: Permaculture is a holistic approach to gardening that seeks to mimic the patterns and relationships found in nature. It emphasizes sustainability, the conservation of resources, and the creation of a self-sustaining ecosystem. Key permaculture principles that can be applied to your medicinal garden include:

- **Observe and Interact**: Spend time in your garden to understand its unique conditions and microclimates. This knowledge will help you select the best locations for your herbs and design your garden layout more effectively.
- **Catch and Store Energy**: Utilize natural resources, such as rainwater and sunlight, to your advantage. Collect rainwater in barrels for irrigation, and position your garden to receive optimal sunlight throughout the day.
- **Use and Value Diversity**: Plant a variety of herbs and companion plants to create a balanced ecosystem that can resist pests and diseases naturally. Diverse plantings also provide habitat for beneficial insects and wildlife.

- **Integrate Rather Than Segregate**: Design your garden so that each element serves multiple functions. For example, a trellis can support climbing plants like **beans** or **cucumbers** while also providing shade for more delicate herbs.
- **Use Edges and Value the Marginal**: The edges of your garden, where different ecosystems meet, are often the most productive areas. Utilize these spaces by planting herbs that can thrive in the transitional conditions, such as **echinacea**, which can tolerate both wet and dry soils.

By applying companion planting and permaculture principles to your medicinal garden, you create a space that is not only beautiful and productive but also resilient and sustainable. This approach allows you to work with nature, rather than against it, resulting in a garden that provides a rich array of medicinal herbs for your family's health and well-being.

Harvesting and Preserving Herbs

Harvesting your herbs at the optimal time is crucial for ensuring they retain the maximum potency of their medicinal properties. For most herbs, this means harvesting in the late morning, after the dew has evaporated but before the sun is at its peak. This timing ensures that the plants are not damp, which could lead to mold during the drying process, yet they still contain a high concentration of essential oils, which are often at their peak due to photosynthesis. When harvesting, use sharp, clean shears or scissors to cut the plants. This minimizes damage and stress to the plants, encouraging healthy regrowth for future harvests. It's important to harvest only the amount you need, leaving enough of the plant to continue its growth cycle.

Once harvested, the method of preserving your herbs plays a significant role in maintaining their therapeutic qualities. Drying is one of the most traditional and effective methods for preserving herbs. To properly dry herbs, tie the stems together and hang them upside down in a warm, dry, and well-ventilated area out of direct sunlight. For herbs with larger leaves or moisture-rich herbs, like mint or basil, a food dehydrator set at a low temperature can be more effective. This method allows for a more controlled drying environment, reducing the risk of mold or mildew spoiling the herbs. Ensure that the herbs are completely dry before storage; any remaining moisture can lead to mold. Once dry, the leaves can be stripped from the stems and stored in airtight containers, labeled with the herb name and date of harvest. Glass jars are preferred for storage as they do not impart any flavors onto the herbs and protect them from light, which can degrade their quality over time.

For those herbs used for their roots, such as dandelion or valerian, the harvesting process is a bit different. These should be dug up in the fall, after the aerial parts of the plant have begun to die back and the plant's energy is concentrated in the roots. Clean the roots thoroughly, removing any soil and debris, and then slice them into thin pieces to promote even drying. Similar to leafy herbs, these can be dried in a dehydrator or air-dried in a well-ventilated space.

Another method for preserving the potency of your herbs is through freezing. This method is particularly useful for herbs that do not dry well, such as basil, chives, or parsley. To freeze herbs, wash and dry them thoroughly, then chop them finely. Spread the chopped herbs on a baking sheet to freeze individually, and once frozen, transfer them to airtight containers or freezer bags. This method preserves the fresh flavor and medicinal properties of the herbs for use in cooking or making fresh herbal remedies throughout the year.

In addition to drying and freezing, making herbal oils and vinegars is an excellent way to preserve the medicinal qualities of your herbs. This involves steeping fresh or dried herbs in high-quality oil or vinegar, allowing the active compounds to infuse into the liquid. These infused oils and vinegars can then be used as bases for salad dressings, marinades, or topical applications, offering a convenient and effective way to incorporate the healing properties of herbs into your daily routine.

By understanding and applying these harvesting and preserving techniques, you can ensure that your home apothecary is well-stocked with potent, high-quality herbs throughout the year. Whether you're making teas, tinctures, salves, or simply using herbs to enhance your cooking, the right harvesting and preservation methods are key to maximizing the effectiveness of your herbal remedies.

Tincturing is another invaluable method for preserving the medicinal properties of herbs. This process involves soaking herbs in a solvent, typically alcohol, to extract the active compounds. Vodka or brandy are commonly used due to their high alcohol content, which effectively extracts and preserves the medicinal qualities of the herbs. To make a tincture, fill a jar one-third to one-half full with dried herbs, then pour in enough alcohol to cover the herbs by at least two inches. Seal the jar and store it in a cool, dark place, shaking it daily for four to six weeks. After this period, strain the liquid through a fine mesh sieve or cheesecloth, squeezing out as much liquid as possible. Store the finished tincture in amber glass dropper bottles for easy use. Tinctures have a long shelf life and offer a convenient, concentrated form of herbal remedy that can be easily administered in precise doses.

Herbal vinegars are also a potent way to capture the essence of herbs, especially for those who prefer a non-alcoholic preservation method. Apple cider vinegar is a popular choice due to its own health benefits, which complement the properties of the herbs. To create an herbal vinegar, pack a clean jar with fresh herbs, then fill the jar with vinegar, ensuring the herbs are completely submerged to prevent mold growth. Seal the jar and let it sit for three to six weeks in a cool, dark place, shaking it occasionally. Strain the vinegar into clean bottles. Herbal vinegars can be used in culinary applications or diluted with water for topical use.

For immediate use, fresh herb pastes offer a way to preserve herbs short-term and enhance the flavor and medicinal properties of meals. Combine fresh herbs with a small amount of oil or water in a food processor to create a paste, which can be frozen in ice cube trays for long-term storage. These cubes can be added directly to soups, stews, or sauces, providing a burst of flavor and health benefits.

Lastly, herbal salts are a simple yet effective way to preserve herbs and add a nutritious boost to dishes. Finely chop fresh herbs and mix them with sea salt, then spread the mixture on a baking sheet to dry. Once dry, store the herbal salt in airtight containers. This method not only extends the life of your herbs but also enriches your diet with their concentrated medicinal properties.

Each of these preservation methods offers a unique way to maintain the integrity and potency of your medicinal herbs, ensuring that you have access to their health benefits year-round. By incorporating a variety of techniques, you can create a comprehensive home apothecary that supports wellness in multiple ways, from culinary enhancements to direct medicinal applications.

Drying and Storing Herbs

To ensure the longevity and potency of your herbs, proper drying and storing techniques are paramount. After harvesting, the next critical step is to **dry your herbs efficiently** to preserve their medicinal qualities. A well-ventilated, dark, and dry area is ideal for this process. Humidity and direct sunlight can degrade the active compounds in herbs, so choosing the right location is crucial. For herbs with high moisture content, such as **mint** or **basil**, using a food dehydrator set between 95°F to 115°F (35°C to 46°C) can expedite the drying process while minimizing the risk of mold or mildew. Ensure herbs are spread out in a single layer on the dehydrator trays to allow for even air circulation.

For those preferring traditional air-drying methods, bundle the herbs loosely with string and hang them upside down. This method works exceptionally well for herbs with lower moisture content, such as **lavender** and **rosemary**. Ensure bundles are not too thick to facilitate air circulation around each stem and leaf. It typically takes 1 to 2 weeks for herbs to dry completely using this method. The herbs are ready when leaves crumble easily between your fingers.

Once dried, the next step is **storing your herbs to maintain their therapeutic properties**. Herbs should be stored in airtight containers away from direct sunlight and heat. Glass jars with tight-fitting lids are ideal as they do not impart any odors or chemicals onto the herbs. Label each container with the herb's name and the date of drying to keep track of freshness. Properly dried herbs can last up to a year if stored correctly, though it's best to use them within six months for maximum potency.

For roots like **dandelion** and **valerian**, after washing and slicing them, lay them out on drying racks or a dehydrator tray. The drying temperature for roots should be slightly higher, around 95°F to 115°F (35°C to 46°C), due to their denser nature. Once dried, store them in airtight containers, similarly to leafy herbs, to protect from moisture and light.

Freezing is another viable option for preserving herbs, especially those that lose their essence when dried, such as **cilantro** and **parsley**. To freeze herbs, wash and pat them dry, chop finely, and spread on a baking sheet to freeze individually. Once frozen, transfer the herbs to freezer bags or containers. This method preserves the fresh taste and some of the medicinal qualities of the herbs for use in cooking and remedies.

Creating an optimal environment for drying and storage is essential. Monitor the humidity and temperature of your drying area regularly, using dehumidifiers or fans if necessary to maintain a dry environment. In humid climates, consider using silica gel packets in your storage containers to absorb any excess moisture that could spoil the herbs.

Remember, the key to preserving the full medicinal value of your herbs lies in the **attention to detail** during the drying and storing processes. By following these precise steps, you ensure that your home apothecary is stocked with high-quality herbs ready for use in natural remedies and culinary creations.

Herbal Seeds and Cuttings

Expanding your medicinal garden through the propagation of seeds and cuttings is a cost-effective and rewarding process that ensures the sustainability of your home apothecary. By carefully selecting and preparing seeds and cuttings from healthy parent plants, you can cultivate a diverse array of herbs tailored to your family's health needs and the specific conditions of your garden.

Seed Selection and Storage: Choose high-quality, non-GMO, and, if possible, organic seeds from reputable suppliers to guarantee the best start for your plants. Pay attention to the seed's viability period, as some herbs have seeds that lose germination capacity quickly. To store seeds, keep them in a cool, dry place away from direct sunlight. Using airtight containers, such as small glass jars with silica gel packets, can help maintain optimal moisture levels and extend the seeds' viability. Label each container with the herb name and the date of collection or purchase for future reference.

Seed Starting Indoors: Starting seeds indoors allows for better control over the germination environment. Use a sterile seed starting mix and shallow trays or pots to sow your seeds. The depth at which you plant the seeds should be approximately twice the size of the seed itself, ensuring not to plant them too deep. Cover the trays with a clear plastic dome or wrap to maintain humidity, and place them in a warm area to encourage germination. A heat mat set to 70°F (21°C) can significantly improve germination rates for warmth-loving herbs. Once seedlings emerge, remove the cover and move the trays to a well-lit area or under grow lights, ensuring they receive at least 16 hours of light daily to prevent leggy growth.

Transplanting Seedlings: When seedlings develop their second set of true leaves, they are ready to be transplanted into individual pots. Handle the delicate seedlings by their leaves rather than their stems to avoid damage. Transplanting them into a slightly larger pot with a high-quality potting mix will provide the nutrients necessary for continued growth. Gradually acclimate seedlings to outdoor conditions over a week before planting them in their final location in the garden to prevent shock.

Propagation by Cuttings: Propagating herbs through cuttings is an efficient way to clone your favorite plants, ensuring a genetically identical copy. Select healthy, non-flowering shoots from the parent plant in the early morning when the plant is fully hydrated. Using a sharp, sterilized knife or scissors, cut a 4-6 inch segment just below a leaf node, where the concentration of growth hormones is highest. Remove the lower leaves, leaving two to four leaves at the top, to reduce moisture loss and focus the plant's energy on root development.

Prepare pots with a mix of half perlite and half peat for optimal drainage and aeration. Dip the cut end of the cutting into a rooting hormone to increase the success rate, then insert it into the prepared potting mix. Water gently to settle the mix around the cutting and cover the pot with a plastic bag or place it in a mini greenhouse to maintain high humidity. Keep the cuttings in a bright, indirect light location and ensure the potting mix remains moist but not waterlogged. Roots typically develop within 4-6 weeks, after which the new plants can be gradually acclimated to outdoor conditions and transplanted into the garden.

Care for New Plants: Whether grown from seeds or cuttings, young plants require careful attention to thrive. Ensure they are watered consistently, keeping the soil moist but not saturated. A balanced, slow-release organic fertilizer can support their growth without overwhelming them with nutrients. Monitor the plants for signs of pests or diseases, treating any issues promptly to prevent spread.

By mastering the techniques of making herbal seeds and cuttings, you can expand your medicinal garden, ensuring a continuous supply of herbs for your family's wellness needs. This practice not only deepens your connection to the healing power of plants but also contributes to the preservation of herbal knowledge and biodiversity for future generations.

Chapter 12: Advanced Herbal Preparations

As we delve into the realm of advanced herbal preparations, it's essential to understand the sophisticated techniques that can amplify the potency and extend the shelf life of herbal remedies. One such technique is the art of **distillation**, a process used to extract essential oils and hydrosols from plants. This method not only captures the essence and therapeutic properties of the herb but also provides a concentrated form that can be used in a variety of applications, from aromatherapy to topical treatments.

Distillation requires specific equipment, namely a still, which can be either purchased as a complete unit or assembled from individual components. The basic principle involves heating the plant material with water or steam, which then carries the volatile compounds through the still. As the steam cools and condenses back into a liquid, it separates into essential oil and hydrosol, with the oil typically floating on top due to its lighter density. This process not only yields highly concentrated essential oils but also hydrosols, which are the water-based solutions that retain the water-soluble compounds of the plant.

For those interested in incorporating distillation into their home apothecary, it's crucial to select the right plants. Not all herbs produce a significant amount of essential oil, and some may require large quantities of plant material to yield even a small amount of oil. Herbs like **lavender**, **peppermint**, and **rosemary** are excellent choices for beginners due to their higher oil content and ease of growing. When harvesting plants for distillation, timing is key; the concentration of essential oils in a plant can vary depending on the time of day, weather conditions, and the plant's growth stage. Typically, harvesting in the morning after the dew has evaporated but before the sun is at its peak will yield the highest concentration of oils.

Safety is another critical aspect of distillation. The process involves heat and potentially flammable substances, so it's important to follow safety guidelines meticulously. Always use the still in a well-ventilated area, keep a fire extinguisher nearby, and never leave the distillation process unattended. Additionally, understanding the properties of the essential oils you're working with is vital, as some can be irritating or harmful if not used correctly.

Another advanced preparation technique is **enfleurage**, a traditional method used to capture the fragrance of flowers that do not yield essential oils through distillation. This process involves spreading a thin layer of fat on a glass frame and then pressing the fresh flowers into the fat. Over time, the fat absorbs the fragrance of the flowers. After several weeks, the fat, now infused with the floral scent, can be used as a solid perfume or further processed to extract the fragrant oil. Enfleurage is a labor-intensive technique but offers a way to preserve the delicate scents of flowers like jasmine, lilac, and rose without using heat, which can alter or destroy their natural fragrance.

As we explore these advanced herbal preparations, it's essential to approach each technique with patience and respect for the traditional knowledge that has been passed down through generations. Whether distilling essential oils or capturing the delicate scent of flowers through enfleurage, these methods allow us to deepen our connection with the plant world and harness the full therapeutic potential of herbs.

Moving beyond distillation and enfleurage, **fermentation** emerges as a transformative technique in the realm of herbal preparations, offering a unique avenue to harness the power of beneficial microbes. This method not only enhances the bioavailability of the herbs' nutrients but also creates probiotic-rich formulations that can support digestive health and boost the immune system. Fermenting herbs involves a simple yet precise process of submerging the plant material in a brine solution or mixing it with a culture starter, then allowing the natural fermentation process to occur over several days or weeks. Herbs like **dandelion**, **nettle**, and **burdock** are particularly well-suited for fermentation, yielding tonics and elixirs that integrate seamlessly into a holistic wellness regimen.

Fermentation requires careful attention to cleanliness and monitoring to ensure the process proceeds without contamination. Using non-chlorinated water, sterilized equipment, and high-quality, organic herbs can significantly reduce the risk of unwanted bacterial growth. The fermentation vessel should be kept in a cool, dark place to facilitate the slow, steady fermentation that develops the desired flavors and medicinal properties. Observing the ferment for signs of activity, such as bubbles or a slight sour aroma, indicates that the process is underway. Once fermentation is complete, the herbal preparation can be strained and stored in the refrigerator to slow further fermentation and preserve its potency.

Solar infusions represent another advanced technique, harnessing the sun's energy to gently extract the medicinal compounds from herbs. This method involves placing herbs in a clear glass jar filled with a carrier oil, such as olive or almond oil, then sealing the jar and placing it in a sunny location for several weeks. The warmth from the sun facilitates a gentle extraction process, resulting in an infused oil that captures the essence and therapeutic properties of the herb. Solar infusions work exceptionally well with herbs like **St. John's wort**, **calendula**, and **chamomile**, producing oils that can be used for massage, skincare, or as a base for further herbal preparations.

The key to successful solar infusions lies in the selection of high-quality carrier oils and herbs, ensuring that the plant material is completely submerged in the oil to prevent mold growth. Rotating the jar daily allows for even exposure to the sun's rays, promoting a more uniform extraction. After the infusion period, the oil is strained through a fine mesh sieve or cheesecloth, and stored in a dark glass bottle to protect it from light degradation. This method not only provides a potent herbal remedy but also embodies the principles of sustainability and simplicity, utilizing natural resources to create healthful preparations.

Advanced herbal preparations, such as distillation, enfleurage, fermentation, and solar infusions, open up a world of possibilities for those seeking to deepen their practice of herbal medicine. Each technique offers a unique way to connect with the healing power of plants, whether through capturing their essential oils, preserving their delicate scents, enhancing their nutritional profile, or extracting their medicinal compounds with the sun's warmth. By embracing these methods, we can create a diverse array of remedies that support health and wellness in a holistic, sustainable manner.

Fermenting Herbal Remedies

Fermenting herbal remedies is a practice that dates back centuries, offering a way to preserve the beneficial properties of herbs while enhancing their nutritional value and bioavailability. The process of fermentation involves the breakdown of the herbs' components by beneficial bacteria, yeasts, and molds, which convert sugars and starches into alcohol or acids. This not only preserves the herbs but also creates compounds with potent health benefits, including probiotics, which are known to support gut health and boost the immune system. To embark on fermenting herbal remedies, it's essential to understand the materials needed, the preparation steps, and the conditions required for successful fermentation.

Materials Needed:
- **Glass Jars:** Choose wide-mouth jars, which allow for easy packing of herbs and removal of the finished product. Ensure the jars are sterilized to prevent contamination.
- **Non-chlorinated Water:** Chlorine can inhibit fermentation, so use filtered or spring water.
- **Sea Salt or Himalayan Pink Salt:** Acts as a preservative and inhibits the growth of unwanted bacteria. Avoid iodized salt as it can halt the fermentation process.
- **Herbs:** Fresh or dried herbs can be used. Popular choices for fermentation include dandelion greens, nettle, and burdock root due to their high nutrient content and health benefits.
- **Starter Culture (optional):** While not always necessary, a starter culture can kickstart the fermentation process. This could be a whey from yogurt or a commercially available fermentation starter.

Preparation Steps:
1. **Prepare the Herbs:** If using fresh herbs, wash them thoroughly to remove any dirt or debris. For dried herbs, ensure they are fully rehydrated by soaking them in non-chlorinated water for several hours or overnight.
2. **Create a Brine:** Dissolve sea salt in non-chlorinated water to create a brine solution. The typical ratio is 1-3 tablespoons of salt per quart of water, depending on the herb's susceptibility to spoilage and the desired taste.
3. **Pack the Jars:** Place the herbs in the sterilized jars, leaving about an inch of space at the top. Pour the brine over the herbs until they are completely submerged. If using a starter culture, add it to the jars according to the package instructions.
4. **Weigh Down the Herbs:** It's crucial that the herbs remain submerged in the brine to prevent mold growth. Use a clean, boiled rock, a fermentation weight, or a small zip-lock bag filled with brine as a weight.

5. **Cover the Jars:** Cover the jars with a cloth and secure it with a rubber band or string. This allows gases produced during fermentation to escape while keeping out contaminants.
6. **Fermentation Period:** Store the jars at room temperature (between 65°F to 75°F) away from direct sunlight. The fermentation period can vary from a few days to several weeks, depending on the herb and the desired potency. Check the jars regularly for signs of fermentation, such as bubbles, and to ensure the herbs remain submerged.

After Fermentation:
Once the desired fermentation period has elapsed, taste the herbs to ensure they have reached the preferred level of sourness. If satisfied, replace the cloth with a tight-fitting lid and store the jars in the refrigerator to drastically slow down the fermentation process. The fermented herbal remedies can now be used as a health supplement, added to meals, or taken as directed for specific health benefits.

Maintenance and Troubleshooting:
- **Mold:** If mold appears on the surface, it's often a result of the herbs not being fully submerged. Remove the moldy parts, and ensure the remaining herbs are fully submerged. If the mold penetrates deeply, it's safest to discard the batch.
- **Odor:** A strong, unpleasant odor can indicate contamination. While a sour or tangy smell is normal, anything resembling spoilage should be discarded.
- **Cloudiness:** It's normal for the brine to become cloudy during fermentation. This is a sign of active fermentation and is not a cause for concern.

Incorporating fermented herbal remedies into your wellness routine can offer numerous health benefits, including improved digestion, enhanced nutrient absorption, and a strengthened immune system. By following these detailed steps and maintaining cleanliness and patience throughout the process, you can successfully ferment a variety of herbs and enjoy their enhanced therapeutic properties.

Herbal Kombuchas and Kvass

Transitioning from the foundational practices of fermentation, we delve into the preparation of herbal kombuchas and kvass, beverages renowned for their probiotic benefits and adaptability to incorporate medicinal herbs. These fermented drinks not only offer a refreshing alternative to water or tea but also serve as vehicles for delivering herbal benefits in a digestible form. The process for creating these beverages, while straightforward, requires precision and attention to detail to ensure both safety and efficacy.

Herbal Kombucha Preparation:
Kombucha, a fermented tea, traditionally combines black or green tea with sugar, water, and a SCOBY (Symbiotic Culture Of Bacteria and Yeast). To infuse this concoction with herbal benefits, one can introduce medicinal herbs during or after the fermentation process.

1. **Brewing the Base:** Begin by brewing a strong herbal tea. Opt for herbs that complement kombucha's natural tanginess, such as ginger for its digestive properties or hibiscus for its high vitamin C content. Use one gallon of purified water to steep approximately 1 cup of dried herbs, ensuring the water is not too hot to preserve the herbs' therapeutic properties.

2. **Adding the SCOBY:** Once the herbal tea cools to room temperature, add the SCOBY and 1 cup of starter tea from a previous batch to prevent unwanted bacteria growth. If incorporating the herbs directly into the SCOBY vessel, ensure they are finely strained to avoid disrupting the SCOBY's structure.

3. **Fermentation:** Cover the brewing vessel with a breathable cloth and secure it with a rubber band. Place the vessel in a warm, dark area where the temperature is consistently between 68°F to 78°F. The fermentation period can range from 7 to 14 days, depending on the desired level of acidity and effervescence.

4. **Flavoring and Bottling:** After the initial fermentation, remove the SCOBY and reserve some liquid for the next batch. At this stage, additional herbal infusions or fresh herbs can be added for a second fermentation, which enhances the kombucha's flavor and carbonation. Bottle the kombucha in clean, airtight bottles, leaving some headspace for carbonation to build. Store the bottles at room temperature for 2 to 3 days before transferring them to the refrigerator to slow fermentation and chill before consumption.

Kvass Preparation:
Kvass, traditionally a Slavic beverage made from rye bread, can be adapted to include a variety of herbs for a nutritious and probiotic-rich drink. The preparation of herbal kvass is simpler and quicker than kombucha, making it an excellent starting point for beginners.

1. **Selecting the Base:** While rye bread is traditional, kvass can be made with fruits, vegetables, or even just herbs. For an herbal kvass, choose robust herbs like mint, lemon balm, or rosemary. Combine these with organic fruits or vegetables if desired, to add layers of flavor.

2. **Preparing the Mixture:** In a large jar, combine about 1/4 cup of sugar with 1 quart of non-chlorinated water, stirring until the sugar dissolves. Add your choice of herbs, and if using, chopped fruits or vegetables. Introduce a slice of sourdough bread or a piece of rye bread as a source of yeast.

3. **Fermentation:** Cover the jar with a cloth and secure it with a rubber band. Place the jar in a warm area, away from direct sunlight, and allow it to ferment for 2 to 5 days. The duration will depend on the ambient temperature and the desired strength of the kvass.

4. **Straining and Storing:** Once fermentation is complete, strain the kvass to remove the solids. Bottle the liquid and refrigerate it. Kvass is best enjoyed chilled and can be consumed within a week for optimal freshness and probiotic content.

Both herbal kombucha and kvass offer a canvas for experimentation with different herbs and flavor profiles. When selecting herbs, consider their therapeutic benefits and how they might complement or enhance the beverage's probiotic qualities. For instance, herbs with natural antibacterial properties, such as thyme or oregano, can be beneficial but should be used judiciously to avoid inhibiting the beneficial bacteria's growth. Similarly, calming herbs like lavender or chamomile can add a relaxing dimension to these traditionally invigorating drinks.

As with all fermented products, cleanliness and attention to the health of the fermentation culture are paramount. Always use sterilized equipment, fresh, high-quality ingredients, and pay close attention to the fermentation environment. The result will be a probiotic-rich beverage that not only tastes delightful but also contributes to the holistic wellness of the family, aligning with the principles of a home apothecary.

Cosmetic Formulations with Herbs

In the realm of **cosmetic formulations with herbs**, creating personalized skincare products allows for a deep connection to the natural world and an understanding of the beneficial properties of plants. The process begins with selecting **high-quality herbs** that target specific skin concerns, such as chamomile for its soothing properties, lavender for its healing effects, or rosemary for its ability to enhance circulation. These herbs can be infused into oils, turned into hydrosols, or dried and powdered for use in various cosmetic formulations.

Herbal Infused Oils:
1. **Select a Carrier Oil:** Choose an oil that suits your skin type. Jojoba oil is great for most skin types due to its similarity to the skin's natural sebum, while coconut oil is preferred for its moisturizing properties, and grapeseed oil is lightweight and suitable for oily skin.
2. **Prepare the Herbs:** Dry the herbs thoroughly to remove any moisture that could cause the oil to go rancid. Once dried, chop or bruise the herbs to increase the surface area for infusion.
3. **Infusion Process:** Combine the herbs and carrier oil in a clean, dry jar. The ratio of herb to oil varies, but a general guideline is 1 part herb to 10 parts oil by volume. Place the jar in a sunny window or a warm place for 4-6 weeks, shaking daily to mix the herbs. For a quicker method, gently heat the oil and herbs in a double boiler for 2-4 hours, ensuring the oil does not overheat.
4. **Strain and Store:** Once the infusion period is complete, strain the oil through a fine mesh sieve or cheesecloth into a clean, dry bottle. Store the infused oil in a cool, dark place.

Herbal Hydrosols:
Creating hydrosols involves distilling fresh herbs, capturing their essential oils and essence in water form. This process requires specialized equipment but yields a gentle, therapeutic product ideal for facial toners or refreshing spritzes.

Herbal Powders for Cosmetics:
1. **Drying Herbs:** Ensure herbs are completely dry to prevent mold in your final product.

2. **Grinding:** Use a coffee grinder or mortar and pestle to grind the herbs into a fine powder.
3. **Sifting:** Sift the powder to remove any large particles for a smooth cosmetic application.
4. **Usage:** Herbal powders can be used as natural colorants or for their therapeutic properties in face masks, makeup, or body powders.

Creating a Simple Herbal Face Mask:
1. **Select Herbs:** Choose herbs that match your skin's needs. For example, green tea powder for antioxidants, rose petal powder for soothing, and bentonite clay for detoxification.
2. **Mix Ingredients:** Combine 1 tablespoon of your chosen herbal powder with enough water, honey, or yogurt to form a paste. For added benefits, include a few drops of an herbal infused oil.
3. **Application:** Apply the mask to clean skin, leaving it on for 10-15 minutes before rinsing with warm water.

Lip Balms with Herbal Infused Oils:
1. **Ingredients:** Combine 2 tablespoons of herbal infused oil with 1 tablespoon of beeswax and 1 tablespoon of shea butter or cocoa butter in a double boiler.
2. **Melting:** Gently heat until the beeswax and butter have melted and are well combined with the oil.
3. **Cooling:** Pour the mixture into clean lip balm tubes or tins and allow to cool completely before capping.

Safety and Testing:
When creating herbal cosmetics, always perform a patch test on a small area of skin to check for adverse reactions. Ensure all containers and tools are sterilized to prevent contamination.

By harnessing the power of herbs, you can create effective, natural skincare products tailored to your family's needs. Whether infusing oils, crafting hydrosols, or incorporating herbal powders, the key is patience and respect for the natural properties of plants. With these techniques, you can bring the healing power of herbs into your daily skincare routine, enhancing wellness and promoting a sustainable lifestyle.

Crafting Herbal Lotions and Creams

Crafting herbal lotions and creams is an advanced yet rewarding aspect of herbal apothecary that allows for the creation of personalized skincare products designed to nourish and heal the skin. This process involves emulsifying water and oils with the addition of herbal extracts to address specific skin concerns. The key to successful formulations lies in understanding the properties of each ingredient and how they interact with each other.

Selecting Base Oils and Butters:
Begin by choosing base oils and butters that align with your skin type and the desired consistency of the final product. For a lighter lotion, grapeseed or almond oil may be ideal, offering quick absorption without leaving a greasy residue. For richer creams, shea butter or cocoa butter provides a dense, moisturizing base

that is particularly beneficial for dry or mature skin. The ratio of oil to water will significantly influence the texture, with higher oil concentrations yielding thicker creams.

Incorporating Herbal Extracts:
Herbal extracts can be added to the oil phase or water phase depending on their solubility. Water-soluble extracts, such as aloe vera juice or rose water, can be included in the water phase, while oil-soluble extracts, like calendula-infused oil or chamomile essential oil, are best added to the oil phase. The choice of herbs should be guided by their therapeutic properties, targeting specific skin issues such as inflammation, dryness, or acne. For instance, green tea extract is renowned for its antioxidant properties, while lavender can soothe irritated skin.

Creating the Emulsion:
The emulsification process is critical in combining the oil and water phases into a stable lotion or cream. This requires an emulsifier, such as beeswax or emulsifying wax, which helps to bind oil and water molecules together. Begin by heating the oil phase and water phase separately in a double boiler until each reaches a temperature of approximately 70°C (158°F). Once both phases are heated, slowly add the oil phase to the water phase while continuously stirring. The mixture should begin to thicken as it cools, forming an emulsion.

Preserving Your Creation:
To ensure the longevity of your herbal lotion or cream, a preservative is necessary. Natural preservatives such as grapefruit seed extract or vitamin E can extend shelf life while adding additional skin benefits. However, it's crucial to research and use the appropriate amount of preservative according to the formulation to prevent microbial growth without compromising the product's integrity.

Adjusting pH:
The pH of skincare products should match the natural pH of the skin, typically around 4.5 to 5.5, to maintain the skin's barrier function. After emulsification, test the pH with strips and adjust if necessary by adding lactic acid to lower the pH or sodium bicarbonate to raise it.

Packaging and Storage:
Once the lotion or cream has cooled and reached the desired consistency, transfer it to sterilized containers. Amber glass jars or bottles can protect the contents from light degradation, preserving the therapeutic qualities of the herbs. Store the product in a cool, dark place to maximize shelf life.

Application and Usage:
Inform users to patch test before applying liberally, especially if essential oils are used, to ensure there is no adverse reaction. Encourage use within the prescribed shelf life for optimal benefits.

By meticulously selecting ingredients, understanding the emulsification process, and adhering to preservation standards, crafting herbal lotions and creams can be a deeply satisfying method to bring the therapeutic power of herbs into everyday skincare routines. This advanced preparation not only enhances the holistic wellness of the family but also empowers individuals with the knowledge to tailor skincare products to their specific needs, embodying the essence of a home apothecary.

Chapter 13: Building Community and Sharing Knowledge

Creating an **Herbal Study Group** can be a transformative way for individuals to deepen their understanding of herbal medicine and build a supportive community. The following steps provide a detailed guide to establishing and maintaining a successful study group:

1. **Define the Purpose and Goals**: Begin by clarifying the group's objectives. Whether it's to learn about herbal remedies for family health, to explore the cultivation of medicinal plants, or to delve into the science behind herbalism, having clear goals will help attract like-minded individuals.

2. **Recruit Members**: Reach out to your local community through social media, community bulletin boards, and local wellness centers. It's beneficial to have members with varying levels of knowledge and experience in herbalism to foster a rich learning environment.

3. **Choose a Meeting Format**: Decide whether meetings will be held in person, online, or a hybrid of both. Consider the frequency of meetings – monthly gatherings can offer a good balance between giving members time to explore topics individually and keeping the momentum going.

4. **Select Study Materials**: Based on the group's interests and goals, choose books, articles, and other resources as study materials. It can be helpful to focus on one book, such as a comprehensive guide to herbal remedies, and supplement it with articles or videos on specific topics of interest.

5. **Plan the Meetings**: Each meeting should have a clear agenda. You might start with a discussion of a chapter from the selected book or an article, followed by a practical demonstration or workshop, such as making a simple herbal remedy or identifying plants on a nature walk.

6. **Guest Speakers and Field Trips**: Inviting experienced herbalists to speak or organizing visits to herbal gardens and apothecaries can provide valuable hands-on learning experiences.

7. **Create a Resource Library**: Encourage members to share books, articles, and online resources. Over time, the group can build a comprehensive library of herbal knowledge.

8. **Document and Share Learning**: Keeping a record of discussions, recipes, and remedies tried by the group can be a valuable resource. Consider creating a shared online document or blog where members can contribute content.

9. **Community Projects**: As the group becomes more established, look for opportunities to engage with the wider community. This could include hosting public workshops, creating a community garden, or volunteering at local health fairs.

10. **Evaluate and Evolve**: Periodically, review the group's goals and activities to ensure they continue to meet the members' needs. Be open to evolving the group's focus or structure as it grows.

Teaching Kids About Herbal Medicine is another vital aspect of building community and sharing knowledge. Engaging children in the world of herbalism can instill an appreciation for nature and teach them valuable skills for natural wellness. Here are some strategies for introducing children to herbal medicine:

- **Herb Gardening**: Start a small garden where children can grow simple herbs like mint, basil, and chamomile. Teach them how to care for the plants and use them in simple recipes or remedies.

- **Herbal Crafts**: Children love hands-on activities. Making herbal sachets, lip balms, or soaps can be a fun way to introduce them to the uses of herbs.

- **Storytelling and Herbal Lore**: Share stories about the history and folklore of plants. Many herbs have fascinating stories that can capture children's imaginations.

- **Nature Walks**: Organize walks in nature to teach children how to identify plants. Use field guides to learn about the plants in your local area.

- **Cooking with Herbs**: Involve children in cooking meals and snacks that incorporate fresh or dried herbs. This is a practical way to teach them about the flavors and health benefits of different herbs.

- **Safety First**: Teach children the importance of safety in herbalism, including which plants are safe to use and the importance of adult supervision when making and using herbal remedies.

By fostering a community of herbal enthusiasts and introducing the next generation to the wonders of plant medicine, we can cultivate a deeper connection to the natural world and empower individuals with the knowledge to care for their health and well-being naturally.

Creating an Herbal Study Group

To ensure the **Herbal Study Group** is both engaging and educational, it's crucial to incorporate a variety of activities that cater to the diverse interests and learning styles of its members. Here are detailed strategies to enrich the group's experience and foster a deeper understanding of herbal medicine:

Developing a Curriculum:

1. **Month-by-Month Themes:** Assign each month a specific theme related to herbal medicine, such as "Herbal Remedies for Digestive Health" or "The Art of Tincture Making." This approach allows members to dive deep into each topic, ensuring a comprehensive understanding.
2. **Skill-Level Grouping:** Recognize the varying skill levels within the group by offering beginner, intermediate, and advanced tracks for some activities. This could mean having separate breakout sessions during meetings or organizing workshops that cater to different experience levels.

Interactive Learning Activities:

1. **Herb of the Month:** Each month, select an herb to study in depth. Members can share research findings, personal experiences, and even bring samples of the herb in various forms, such as dried, tinctures, or salves.
2. **Recipe Swap:** Encourage members to share their favorite herbal recipes, whether it's a medicinal syrup, a beauty product, or a culinary delight. This activity not only promotes sharing of knowledge but also celebrates the versatility of herbs.
3. **Plant Identification Walks:** Organize seasonal walks in local natural areas or members' gardens to practice identifying herbs and other medicinal plants in the wild. This hands-on experience is invaluable for developing practical skills in herbalism.

Workshops and Demonstrations:

1. **Guest Herbalists:** Invite local herbalists to conduct workshops on specific topics, such as wildcrafting ethics, herbal extraction methods, or creating herbal first aid kits. These experts can offer insights beyond the basic curriculum and inspire members with their depth of knowledge.
2. **DIY Herbal Products:** Regularly schedule workshops where members can learn to make their own herbal products, such as lip balms, salves, or herbal teas. Provide a list of materials needed in advance so members can come prepared or contribute to the supplies.

Discussion and Reflection:

1. **Book Club:** Select herbalism-related books for the group to read and discuss. This could be a comprehensive herbal guide, historical accounts of herbal medicine, or contemporary herbal wellness literature. Discussions can be held during meetings or in an online forum for those unable to attend in person.
2. **Case Studies:** Present hypothetical or anonymized real-life scenarios where herbal remedies could be applied. Members can discuss possible herbal approaches, considering factors such as contraindications, dosage, and preparation methods.

Community Engagement:

1. **Herbal Garden Project:** Collaborate on creating a community herbal garden. This project can serve as a practical learning tool for cultivation techniques and as a source of herbs for the group's use.

2. **Public Education:** Plan and host public workshops or talks on herbal wellness topics. This not only serves as a learning experience for members but also promotes herbal medicine within the wider community.

Online Platform for Resource Sharing:
1. **Digital Library:** Create a digital repository of herbalism resources, including articles, videos, and recipes. This can be a shared drive or a private online forum where members can upload and access information.
2. **Discussion Board:** Maintain an active online discussion board where members can post questions, share discoveries, and offer support to one another outside of regular meetings.

By implementing these strategies, the **Herbal Study Group** will not only be a source of knowledge and skill development but also a vibrant community that celebrates the rich traditions and potential of herbal medicine. Through diverse learning activities, hands-on workshops, and community engagement, members can deepen their understanding of herbalism while contributing to the group's collective wisdom and the broader community's well-being.

Teaching Kids Herbal Medicine

Creating engaging and educational experiences for children in the realm of herbal medicine can be both rewarding and fun. By incorporating interactive activities and hands-on learning, children can gain a foundational understanding of plants and their uses in a way that resonates with their innate curiosity about the natural world. Here are some detailed strategies for teaching kids about herbal medicine:

Interactive Herbal Storytelling: Choose books or create stories that weave together the lore, history, and science of plants and herbs. Focus on tales that highlight the role of plants in different cultures and ecosystems. For instance, tell the story of how Native Americans used echinacea for its healing properties or how lavender has been used throughout history for its calming effects. Use vivid descriptions and encourage questions to deepen their engagement.

Herbal Art Projects: Combine creativity with learning by organizing art projects centered around herbs. One idea is to have children press flowers and leaves from safe, non-toxic herbs to create natural art pieces. Another is to use herbal dyes made from beetroot, turmeric, or spinach to paint pictures, teaching them about the colors and properties of different herbs.

Sensory Exploration: Organize a sensory garden or a series of pots with various herbs that children can touch, smell, and taste under supervision. Include herbs with distinctive scents like mint, lemon balm, and rosemary, and those with interesting textures. Guide them through the process of gently rubbing the leaves between their fingers to release the aromas, explaining the uses and benefits of each herb.

Simple Herbal Preparations: Demonstrate how to make simple herbal preparations such as teas, lemon balm ice cubes, or lavender sachets. Use this opportunity to discuss the importance of dosage and safety, emphasizing that even natural substances must be used with care. Provide each child with their own set of ingredients and supervise closely as they learn to measure, mix, and prepare their herbal creations.

Garden to Table: If possible, involve children in growing a selection of easy-to-care-for herbs such as basil, parsley, and cilantro. Guide them through the process from planting seeds to harvesting. Then, incorporate these herbs into cooking lessons, where children can learn to make simple, healthy dishes or snacks that highlight the flavor and nutritional benefits of fresh herbs.

Herbal Science Experiments: Engage children with simple science experiments that illustrate the properties of herbs. For example, create a natural pH indicator using red cabbage and show how it changes color with different substances. Explain the basic science behind why some herbs are used for digestion, sleep, or healing wounds, linking it to the chemical compounds found in plants.

Herbal Scavenger Hunts: Organize scavenger hunts in safe, outdoor areas where children can search for specific plants or herbs. Use this activity to teach them about plant identification, ecological relationships, and the importance of conservation. Provide them with a checklist of plants to find, along with pictures and descriptions to help them identify each one.

Safety and Ethics Discussion: Incorporate discussions about the ethical harvesting of plants and the importance of conservation. Teach them about the concept of sustainable sourcing and why it's important not to overharvest wild plants. Discuss the safety aspects of herbal medicine, emphasizing the need to consult with a knowledgeable adult before using any plant medicinally.

By integrating these activities into your approach to teaching kids about herbal medicine, you can foster a deep appreciation for the natural world and empower them with knowledge that promotes a healthy, sustainable lifestyle. Through hands-on learning and interactive experiences, children can develop a foundational understanding of how plants can support wellness in a way that is both fun and educational.

Chapter 14: Ethical Wildcrafting and Sustainability

Ethical wildcrafting practices are essential for the sustainability of medicinal plant populations and the health of our ecosystems. When wildcrafting, it's crucial to follow guidelines that support the regeneration of wild plants and respect their natural habitats. Begin by researching and understanding the **status of the plants** you intend to harvest. Some species may be endangered or protected, making it illegal or unethical to wildcraft. Utilize resources like the United Plant Savers' "At-Risk" list to identify these plants. Always obtain **permission** before harvesting on private land or in protected areas.

When you've identified a safe and legal area for wildcrafting, practice **mindful harvesting** techniques to ensure plants can continue to grow and propagate. This includes:

1. **Harvesting no more than 10%** of the plants in a given area to avoid overharvesting. This percentage can be even lower for rare or slow-growing species.
2. **Using clean, sharp tools** to make precise cuts that will heal quickly and minimize damage to the plant.
3. **Harvesting at the right time of day and season** for each plant to ensure the highest medicinal quality and to support the plant's lifecycle. For example, leaves are often best harvested in the morning after dew has evaporated but before the sun is too intense, while roots are typically harvested in the fall when the plant's energy is stored below ground.
4. **Respecting the surrounding environment** by not trampling other plants, disturbing wildlife, or leaving trash behind.

Propagation efforts can further support sustainability. Consider planting seeds of the wild plants you harvest or participating in restoration projects to replenish native plant populations. This can be as simple as scattering seeds in appropriate areas during the right season or as involved as growing plants to a transplantable size before reintroducing them to the wild.

Documenting your harvest locations and methods can help you track the health of plant populations over time and refine your practices. Keep a journal of when, where, and how you harvest, including any observations about the abundance of plants and the condition of their habitat. This record-keeping can be invaluable for personal use and can contribute to broader efforts to monitor and conserve medicinal plant populations.

Educating others about ethical wildcrafting and the importance of plant conservation is another critical component. Share your knowledge and practices with fellow herbalists, community groups, and through social media to raise awareness. Hosting workshops or leading wildcrafting walks with an emphasis on sustainability can empower more people to act as stewards of their local plant communities.

Finally, **supporting ethical and sustainable sources** of medicinal plants, whether by purchasing from responsible wildcrafters or choosing companies that prioritize sustainability in their sourcing, reinforces the market for sustainably harvested herbs. This economic encouragement can help shift practices on a larger scale towards more sustainable and ethical approaches to plant medicine.

By adhering to these principles, we can ensure that our practice of wildcrafting not only provides us with the medicinal plants we need but also contributes to the health and vitality of the ecosystems we depend on. Through mindful engagement with the natural world, we sustain the plants that sustain us, fostering a reciprocal relationship that can last for generations.

Responsible Foraging Practices

Responsible foraging practices are not only about knowing which plants to harvest but also understanding how to do so in a way that ensures their sustainability for future generations. When foraging, always carry a field guide specific to the region you are in. This guide should provide detailed information on plant identification, including photographs, descriptions, and the habitats where plants are likely to be found. Before harvesting any plant, confirm its identity using at least two sources to avoid mistaking it for a similar-looking but potentially harmful species.

Harvesting Techniques:

1. **Leaves and Flowers:** Use scissors or garden shears to cut leaves and flowers, leaving enough of the plant intact to ensure its continued growth. Aim to take only the top third of the plant or less, depending on its abundance and regrowth rate.
2. **Roots:** When harvesting roots, be especially mindful of the plant's ability to regenerate. Use a small trowel or digging fork to gently unearth the root, taking care to disturb as little of the surrounding soil and plant life as possible. Only harvest roots from areas where the plant is abundant, and always replant a portion of the root back into the soil to help ensure the plant's return next season.
3. **Seeds:** Collecting seeds requires patience and timing. Wait until the seeds are fully matured but before they have dispersed. Use envelopes or paper bags to collect seeds, labeling each with the date and location of collection. Share excess seeds with fellow foragers or consider planting them in suitable locations to encourage growth.

Foraging Ethics:

- **Respect Private Property:** Always obtain permission before foraging on private land. Many landowners are willing to allow foraging if asked, but trespassing can damage relationships with the community and potentially lead to legal consequences.

- **Avoid Overharvesting:** Be conscious of how much you are taking from any given area and limit your harvest to ensure plants can regenerate. A good rule of thumb is never to take more than 10% of the available plants in any given area, and even less for rare or slow-growing species.
- **Consider the Ecosystem:** Understand the role each plant plays in its ecosystem before deciding to harvest. Some plants may be crucial for local wildlife, providing food or habitat. Removing these plants can have a negative impact on the ecosystem's health.
- **Leave No Trace:** Practice the principles of Leave No Trace by minimizing your impact on the environment. Stick to established trails to avoid trampling undergrowth and habitats, and carry out any trash you bring in or find.

Safety Considerations:
- **Personal Safety:** Always let someone know where you are going and when you plan to return, especially if foraging in remote areas. Carry a basic first aid kit, water, and a cell phone for emergencies.
- **Plant Safety:** Be aware of the potential for allergic reactions and ensure that any plant you plan to consume is safe and has been correctly identified. Start with small quantities to test for personal sensitivities or adverse reactions.

Sustainable Use of Foraged Items:
- **Processing and Preservation:** Process and preserve foraged items promptly to maximize their usefulness and minimize waste. Drying, canning, and freezing are all effective methods for extending the shelf life of foraged goods.
- **Sharing the Bounty:** Share surplus foraged items with friends, family, or community members interested in natural remedies and wild foods. This not only distributes the benefits of foraging but also fosters a sense of community and shared responsibility for local ecosystems.

By adhering to these responsible foraging practices, foragers can enjoy the bounty of nature while contributing to the preservation and health of the environment. Through mindful engagement with the natural world, we can ensure that these resources remain abundant and accessible for future generations.

Conserving Herbal Populations

Conserving herbal populations requires a multifaceted approach, integrating knowledge of ecology, plant biology, and sustainable harvesting practices. To ensure that medicinal plants remain abundant and healthy for future generations, it's crucial to adopt strategies that support their growth and reproduction. Here are specific, actionable steps to conserve herbal populations:

Select Native Plants for Your Garden: Focus on planting native species in your home garden. Native plants are adapted to the local climate and soil conditions, requiring less water and care than non-native species. They also provide essential habitat for local wildlife, including pollinators which are crucial for the reproduction of many medicinal plants. Research the native plants of your region and select those known for their medicinal properties. For example, if you live in the Northeastern United States, consider planting echinacea, goldenseal, and black cohosh, all of which have medicinal uses and are native to the area.

Participate in Seed Exchange Programs: Engage with local gardening clubs or online communities that focus on medicinal plants. Seed exchange programs allow you to diversify the genetic pool of your medicinal plants, which can increase their resilience to diseases and environmental stresses. By sharing seeds, you're also contributing to the spread of medicinal plant populations, which can help counteract the effects of overharvesting in the wild.

Implement Companion Planting: Companion planting is a method that involves growing different plants together to benefit each other. Many medicinal plants can act as natural pest deterrents, improve soil health, and enhance the growth and flavor of other plants. For instance, planting garlic near roses can help deter pests, while marigolds can attract beneficial insects that prey on pests. By carefully selecting companion plants, you can create a healthier ecosystem in your garden that supports the growth of medicinal plants.

Use Organic Gardening Practices: Avoid the use of chemical pesticides and fertilizers, which can harm the soil microbiome and pollinators. Instead, opt for organic gardening practices that enhance soil fertility and plant health. Composting kitchen scraps and yard waste can provide rich, nutrient-dense soil for your plants without the need for chemical fertilizers. Additionally, using natural pest control methods, such as introducing beneficial insects or using plant-based pesticides, can protect your medicinal plants without harming the environment.

Educate Your Community: Share your knowledge about the importance of conserving medicinal plants with your community. Host workshops or create informational materials on how to grow and care for medicinal plants, emphasizing the importance of sustainable practices. Encourage others to plant native medicinal plants in their gardens and to participate in seed exchange programs. By raising awareness, you can inspire collective action towards the conservation of medicinal plant populations.

Support Conservation Organizations: Many organizations are dedicated to the conservation of medicinal plants and their habitats. By supporting these organizations, whether through donations, volunteering, or advocacy, you can contribute to larger-scale efforts to protect medicinal plants. These organizations often engage in habitat restoration, research, and policy advocacy, which are all crucial for the long-term conservation of medicinal plants.

By integrating these practices into your gardening and community engagement, you can play a significant role in conserving herbal populations. Sustainable gardening practices, combined with a commitment to education and support for conservation efforts, can ensure that medicinal plants continue to thrive for generations to come.

Conclusion

Embracing a holistic approach to family wellness through the establishment of a home apothecary is a transformative journey that empowers individuals and families to take charge of their health using ancient natural remedies. The process of learning, preparing, and utilizing these remedies fosters a deep connection with nature, encourages self-reliance, and promotes a sustainable lifestyle that benefits both the individual and the planet. By integrating the wisdom of herbal medicine into daily life, families can experience profound improvements in health, well-being, and overall quality of life.

Creating a home apothecary is more than just assembling a collection of herbs and remedies; it's about cultivating a mindset of proactive health care and a lifestyle that prioritizes natural wellness. This involves educating oneself about the properties and uses of various herbs, understanding the body's natural healing processes, and developing the skills to prepare and apply herbal remedies effectively. It also means adopting practices that support health beyond the physical, including stress management, nutritional adjustments, and regular physical activity, all of which are complementary to the use of herbal medicine.

The journey towards establishing a holistic family home apothecary is ongoing and evolves with time. As individuals gain more knowledge and experience, they become more attuned to the needs of their bodies and their families, enabling them to customize and refine their approach to herbal medicine. This personalization is key to creating a truly effective home apothecary that reflects the unique health needs and wellness goals of each family.

In addition to the personal health benefits, establishing a home apothecary also contributes to the preservation of herbal medicine traditions. By learning about and utilizing ancient remedies, individuals play a role in keeping this valuable knowledge alive and accessible for future generations. This not only enriches the individual's understanding of natural medicine but also supports the broader goal of maintaining biodiversity and ecological balance.

As the practice of herbal medicine regains its rightful place in modern health care, the role of the home apothecary becomes increasingly important. It serves as a testament to the power of nature to heal and nurture, and a reminder of the wisdom inherent in traditional healing practices. Through the conscientious use of herbal remedies, families can enjoy enhanced health and well-being while contributing to the sustainability of natural resources and the preservation of herbal knowledge.

The path to creating a holistic family home apothecary is both rewarding and challenging, requiring dedication, patience, and a willingness to learn. It is a journey that not only transforms the health of individuals and families but also deepens their connection to the natural world. As more people embrace this holistic approach to wellness, the collective impact on public health, environmental sustainability, and the preservation of herbal traditions promises to be profound.

For those embarking on the venture of establishing a home apothecary, the selection of herbs and remedies is just the beginning. A deeper understanding of each herb's properties, the ailments it can address, and the best ways to harness its benefits is essential. This knowledge enables the creation of a personalized apothecary stocked with remedies tailored to the specific health needs and wellness goals of each family member. Furthermore, mastering the art of remedy preparation—from tinctures and salves to teas and poultices—enhances the efficacy of the home apothecary and ensures that remedies are readily available when needed.

Engagement with the community and sharing knowledge about herbal remedies can amplify the benefits of a home apothecary. Organizing workshops, participating in local herb walks, and joining herbal medicine forums online can provide valuable learning opportunities and foster a sense of community among those interested in natural wellness. These activities not only enhance one's own understanding but also contribute to a collective pool of knowledge, supporting the wider adoption of herbal medicine practices.

Sustainability is a core principle of the home apothecary, guiding not only the selection and use of herbs but also the sourcing of supplies. Prioritizing locally grown herbs, engaging in ethical wildcrafting, and supporting suppliers who practice sustainable farming are all ways to ensure that the home apothecary contributes to the health of the planet as well as the individual. This mindful approach to sourcing also connects individuals more deeply with their local ecosystem, encouraging a greater appreciation for the natural resources available in one's own backyard.

Incorporating technology can further enhance the home apothecary experience. Digital resources such as apps for plant identification, online courses on herbal medicine, and virtual communities of herbalists provide access to a wealth of information and support. These tools can help individuals identify local medicinal plants, learn new remedy preparation techniques, and connect with experienced practitioners, enriching the home apothecary journey with a blend of traditional wisdom and modern convenience.

Ultimately, the creation of a holistic family home apothecary is an act of empowerment. It represents a commitment to taking control of one's health and well-being through natural means, fostering a lifestyle that values prevention, nurtures healing, and respects the interconnectedness of humans and the natural world. As families grow in their knowledge and practice of herbal medicine, they not only enhance their own health but also contribute to a larger movement towards sustainable living and holistic wellness. This movement, grounded in ancient traditions yet adapted for the modern world, holds the promise of a healthier future for all.